# THE ICE AGE

Luke Williams is an Australian journalist. He has previously worked as a reporter and broadcaster at ABC radio. His written work has been published in *The Sydney Morning Herald*, *The Saturday Paper*, *Brisbane Times*, *Crikey*, *The Global Mail*, *The Weekend Australian*, and *Eureka Street*. In 2013 he was nominated for a Human Rights Media Award for a long-form investigative piece in *The Global Mail*, and in 2014 his article on ice addiction, 'Life as a Crystal Meth Addict', was a finalist in the Walkley Awards for Excellence in Journalism.

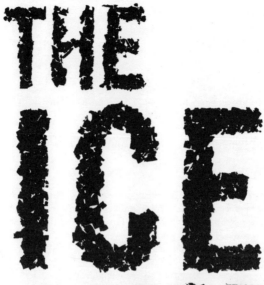

# THE ICE AGE

A JOURNEY INTO CRYSTAL-METH ADDICTION

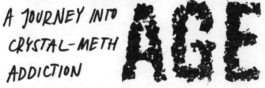

# LUKE WILLIAMS

SCRIBE

*Melbourne • London*

Scribe Publications
18–20 Edward St, Brunswick, Victoria 3056, Australia
2 John St, Clerkenwell, London, WC1N 2ES, United Kingdom

First published by Scribe 2016
This edition published 2017

Earlier versions of parts of this manuscript have appeared in various
publications, including *The Saturday Paper*, *Good Weekend*, and SBS Online.

Typeset in 11.5/15 pt Adobe Garamond Pro by the publishers
Printed and bound in the UK by CPI Group (UK) Ltd, Croydon CR0 4YY

Scribe Publications is committed to the sustainable use of natural resources
and the use of paper products made responsibly from those resources.

A CiP entry for this title is available from the National Library of Australia

9781925106848 (Australian edition)
9781925228922 (UK edition)
9781925307115 (e-book)

scribepublications.com.au
scribepublications.co.uk

# CONTENTS

Author's note     vii

Prologue     1
One: Ice monsters     11
Two: Panic!     35
Three: Converging paths     63
Four: The hazardous bush     85
Five: Rise and fall     111
Six: Every creature has its soft spots     139
Seven: Ridgey didge     165
Eight: Wheeling and dealing     183
Nine: Understanding the lure of crystal meth     205
Ten: Into the Vortex     217
Eleven: Parents and thieves     235
Twelve: The devil     253
Thirteen: Winter     275
Fourteen: Bundaberg     291
Fifteen: Two steps forward, one step back     309
Sixteen: Beyond excess     333

Select bibliography     361
Acknowledgements     367

# AUTHOR'S NOTE

I HAVE DONE my best to recreate events, locales, and conversations from my memories of them, and from my notes. I have in many instances changed the names of individuals, and may also have changed some identifying characteristics and details.

I have recalled the events in this book to the best of my ability, and with the best of intentions. However, at the time of experiencing them, and occasionally at the time of writing about them, I was affected by drugs. At other times, as I recount in the pages that follow, I was experiencing drug-induced psychosis.

As a result, it may be that other peoples' memories of these events will differ from my own.

# Prologue

02/05/2014 12:06

From: Luke Williams

Matt, I wanted to ask you something. I have growing extra-sensory powers since I have started The Journey and have been practising telepathy, I just wanted to see if you or anybody you know have been sending me messages.

02/05/2014 12:08

From: Matt F

Not that I know of.

THE CHEMICAL N-METHYL-1-PHENYL-PROPAN-2-AMINE $(C_{10}H_{15}N)$ better known as 'crystal meth' or 'ice', is a highly addictive drug that has been linked to murder, violence, savage sadism, and woeful child-neglect. It's a drug that feels better than sex; a drug made in Nigeria, Iran, Thailand, and in our own kitchen sinks, which is often sent here from southern China. Meth is the world's strongest stimulant.

Crystal methamphetamine was created in 1919. Thereafter it

was sold in pharmacies to treat depression, fatigue, and obesity. It was also used in the military for performance enhancement in several major wars. It was made more or less completely illegal throughout the western world in the 1970s as the result of a particular UN convention. Since then, the black market for crystal meth has grown rapidly. By the 1980s, crystal-meth production and distribution was dominated by American biker gangs, who then joined up with a Mexican cartel, who in turn provided factories to manufacture meth and its precursors.

Powdered meth (also known as speed) has been available in Australia since the mid-1990s, but rates of meth use really started to increase around 2001 — when Asian illicit-drug crime gangs based in the Golden Triangle wound back their heroin production and started producing meth. The gangs appeared to see meth as a more reliable source of income than heroin because the former would not be affected by increasingly unstable weather.

While researching a story about crystal meth in early 2014, I became addicted to the drug, and began using it heavily. I rapidly descended into psychosis.

During that time, I would sometimes send people online messages and emails.

## Correspondence with my Aunty

Date: 02/03/14
Subject: My Mum has got dementia
To: AnneXX@yahoo.com.au
From: Luke Williams
Aunty Anne. I know we haven't spoken in over 10 years. Please I need to talk to you. I know we haven't spoken in a long time, but I need to tell you how much I miss having your family in my life. Also, I need to talk to you about my

Mum, I think she might be dying of dementia. I am very
worried about her. I had somebody try to bash me the other
day and I rang my parents. They didn't believe me and said
I was on drugs and hung up on me and I was very scared. I
am not on any drugs. They keep on using that as an excuse
so they don't have to face up to the issues I had growing up.
Luke

Date: 08/03/14
Re: My Mum has got dementia
To: Luke Williams
From: AnneXX@yahoo.com.au
Luke, I just spoke to your Mum, she is very worried that
you are using drugs. Don't believe that Janet has dementia
in any form. I think you probably think that because of the
drugs you are taking. She also mentioned you have been
threatening to kill your father, and that you left over 20
threatening messages on her phone the other day. I don't
know what to suggest. I think you need help urgently.
Aunty Anne
XXX

Unlike cocaine or heroin, which come from plants, meth is a
wholly synthetic drug. Meth is commonly manufactured in
illegal, hidden laboratories. Common ingredients include cold
and flu tablets, battery acid, drain cleaner, and lantern fuel. Some
of the meth that is used in Australia is made in 'backyard labs',
and often by individual users in their own sinks and bathtubs.
In recent times, an increasing proportion of Australia's crystal
meth has been produced overseas, usually smuggled in through
air cargo shipped from China and Hong Kong.

Drug manufacturers are getting better at creating purer,
stronger meth. The popularity of the drug on the black market

meant that a diverse range of international crime gangs got on board to produce and distribute the drug. A more potent variety of crystallised meth began to flood Australia's illicit-drug market in 2011, and harms caused by crystal meth have been rising all over the nation ever since. User deaths, arrests, homicides, and hospital admissions have all been rising sharply.

Crystal meth is highly addictive, and in Australia it is relatively cheap and easy to obtain. For $50 you can buy a high that lasts for up to twenty-four hours. In low doses, methamphetamine can cause a heightened mood as well as increased alertness, concentration, and energy. At higher doses, it can induce obsessive behaviour, aggressive behaviour, homicidal ideation, psychosis, heart attacks, and cerebral haemorrhages.

It is believed that crystal meth (like ecstasy and LSD) causes a rise in a user's serotonin levels when they first take it. These serotonin levels drop sharply when you are withdrawing from the drug, but during the high—and contrary to popular belief—a person on crystal meth can actually be extremely nice.

**Email to my estranged ex (he never replied)**

Dear Nats,
I know we had a big, bad break up a few years ago. I know we haven't spoken since. But I just want to let you know that I harbour no ill-feeling toward you, and I think you are a wonderful person.
And don't forget what an excellent hairdresser you are—your styles are always years ahead of trend.
If you ever need any help with anything let me know.
Luke
X

As my meth addiction grew, I began obsessing over Nathaniel all the time, and began to feel more and more as if it was my fault that we broke up. I felt that we should be back together again.

Over time, I believed he was living near me, sending me telepathic messages, and then that people who visited the house were him in disguise and that people had been hiding this information from me. In particular, a girl who I swore was Nate was sleeping with one of my roommates, and I became enraged with envy at times—I felt homicidal toward him—because I believed he had stolen my ex, and then made him have a sex change.

**Correspondence with a former triple j work colleague I hadn't spoken with in a long time**

One of the key affects of meth is that it floods the brain with dopamine.

Dopamine plays an important role in how the brain experiences and interprets pleasure, motivation, and reward. Dopamine also leads to psychotic symptoms, similar to those that someone with paranoid schizophrenia goes through when they are unwell.

One of the most common forms of psychosis I experienced was delusions of reference—from the outset, meth can make you very self-absorbed. I would google myself and find blogs written by people with the same name, and I would have a recurring delusion that these blogs were parodies of me set up by people I used to work with—as you can see from the correspondence below:

15/02/2014

From: Luke Williams

Kate, people are making fun of me everywhere. There is a blog named Luke Williams which has been set up by people to ridicule me and the way I write.

From: Kate Spears

Are you sure you're not reading into things the wrong way? How are you feeling?

From: Luke Williams

No Kate, people are making fun of me all over the internet. People are using my name and sending me in blogs and videos. It's because I have been such a nasty, vindictive person all my life. Somebody has even made an entire parody of me, a guy who reckons he is 'Luke Williams' has made this ted-ex video.

From: Kate Spears

Mate that's a different Luke Williams. You have a very very common name. Not everyone on the internet named Luke Williams is you. You are having a psychotic episode where you think everything is related to you when its not. Go for a walk, get some sunshine, get off the internet, I think you are reading things the wrong way.

The other frequent delusion I had was that there was a paedophile ring operating in my suburb, that my roommates were in on it, that the headquarters were located at the local Coffee Club, and that it was my purpose in life to expose it. Then, at other times, I had positive delusions — such as the belief that something mystical was happening in my life, and that my crystal-meth use played no role in these feelings.

**Correspondence with a guy I'd met in a nightclub three weeks earlier**

02/05/2014
From: Luke Williams
Hi Matt, it was great meeting you in Sydney last month—you and your friends were all very welcoming. I just wanted to tell you—and please don't freak out about this—I have been using crystal meth.

It's actually part of a thing called The Journey. I suspect you might have something to do with this, given your interest in mysticism.

I am onto something good, I know it. I have had a couple of 'episodes' and some horrible memories came out and now I feel so confident and free. I really feel like I am becoming a better, kinder, more open person through The Journey.

02/05/2014 12:05
From: Matt F
Hey Luke, Thanks for the message, Is everything okay? Do you want to talk on the phone later this arvo?

02/05/2014 12:06
From: Luke Williams
Yes please, thanks, because I wanted to ask you something. I have growing extra-sensory powers since I have started The Journey and have been practising telepathy, I just wanted to see if you or anybody you know have been sending me messages.

02/05/2014 12:08
From: Matt F
Not that I know of.

02/05/2014 12:06
From: Luke Williams
Okay. Do you know anybody who practises witchcraft, because I think one of your friends has cast a spell on me. I feel like I am under some sort of spell, and it is making me change in some way.

**Correspondence with my mum**

More than 500,000 Australians take powdered and crystallised meth each year, and between 10 per cent and 20 per cent of those are considered to be either abusers of the drug or addicted to it.

The Victorian and Northern Territory parliaments have both held official inquiries into the crystal-meth problem in their communities. The New South Wales Police Commissioner, Andrew Scipione, has said that if we don't adequately address this problem, it's not an overstatement to say that '[crystal meth] could bring us to our knees as a nation'. Gordian Fulde, the head of emergency at Sydney's St Vincent Hospital, says he finds ice users to be the 'most violent human beings I have seen'. In New South Wales, Australia's most populated state, places such as western New South Wales, Nowra, and Mt Druitt are showing signs of having the highest rates of harm caused by meth. While Western Australia has the highest per-capita meth use, Queensland remains Australia's meth-production capital, and crystal-meth use is increasing across all of South Australia and Tasmania.

There have been extraordinarily long waiting lists to get into rehabs and even to see a drug counsellor in many parts of the country—particularly in regional Victoria and the Australian

Capital Territory. This often leaves users in the hands of family members, who are in turn at a loss as to what to do.

Date: 02/06/14
Subject: Please Help
To: janetwilliamsXX@dodo.com.au
From: Luke Williams
Mum,
I am sorry about everything. Please help me, please I am scared.
Please help me.

# Chapter One

# Ice monsters

I SMELT LIKE a dead pig. My hair looked awful. There were dark rings around my eyes, and dog-shit on my teeth. Smithy wouldn't stop masturbating. Daytime television was blaring all over the house—*NYPD Blue*, *Hawaii-50*, *JAG*. There were never-ending television programs running in our heads, too. Smithy's sexual fantasies were particularly vivid and enduring, full of highly skilled method actors who knew his tastes perfectly well—right down to the costumes, and the lack of dialogue and backstory. There were all kinds of different people in guest-star roles, in long-running plots, doing whatever Smithy wanted and liking whatever he liked: saucy librarians, the people next-door, a horny, rough-necked bisexual couple, and so on.

Smithy was in a sexual-fantasy world that released him from his most pressing, most unpleasant, and most urgent real-life problems as the father of three kids. But on this day, these fantasies were being used for another, more deliberate purpose—distraction and metaphor. Things seemed normal—dare I say, *suspiciously* normal. I'd just worked out that Smithy had been conspiring to kill me for months, and that my parents were paying him to do it.

Here's how it panned out: it was a bright Tuesday autumn afternoon, and we were in the middle of a meth binge. Just another day in Pakenham, really. Smithy was wearing a red T-shirt and white tracksuit pants; I was in my tartan 'daytime' pyjamas. We were sitting in the lounge room of Smithy's neat, new, spotlessly clean home. Three bedrooms, two living areas, furniture assembled around televisions, a 1997 computer with no internet, and smooth white walls, one with a framed picture of the 1991 Collingwood football team posing and smiling as if they were in a school photo.

As usual, the curtains were closed, and the scent of bleach (and bong smoke) was in the air. Clean carpets, filthy minds: when Smithy wasn't cleaning, he was usually masturbating, for six to eight hours at a time, stopping only to pull a bong. Having visitors rarely stopped him.

Smithy masturbated so much because he shot up meth. I suppose you could call him a junkie. He was also an occasional drug-dealer, a long-time friend, and a full-time house cleaner—a cricket-loving, needle-using, dole-bludging Collingwood fan. He'd adapted poorly to new technology, feminism, and the demand for high-skilled workers—in fact, I could probably save some time by just referring to him as 'Smithy from the 80s', because in many ways it's as if he never left them. A graduate of rehab and the army, he had also, about three years earlier, graduated from 'truckie speed' to using meth full-time. He had a track mark that looked like a chunky, purple birthmark.

He was constantly pulling shady little scams to get by, and he must have sensed the opportunity for another one a few weeks earlier when I'd pissed my parents off. He and my dad must have discussed the plot at length over the phone at night, while I was in bed. My dad would hand over $5,000 now, and then another $5,000 when the deed was done.

Smithy had been dropping hints all day that there was a plot to kill me. He'd been yelling at me about the state of my skin, my odour, the fact I hadn't shaved in over a month, and my tendency to put my plates away in the bookshelf instead of in the sink. What this *meant*, though, was that Mum and Dad were paying him to slip me small, untraceable bits of arsenic mixed with doses of crystal meth. They knew full well that I had a history of drug addiction, loved living in a fantasy world, and that I couldn't say no to the world's most powerful stimulant—the perfect potion to hide your poison in. Smithy had been giving my dad regular updates on my 'progress' for weeks, and every time I left the room, my roommates would snicker. The plan was all falling into place—I had been so off-my-face for the past month, I hadn't even noticed what was going on.

I knew that arsenic works by blocking the molecules your body's cells need to perform their tasks. Eventually, arsenic kills by causing haemorrhaging, destroying enough cells to cause multi-system organ failure. So the arsenic poison had been building up in my liver and intoxicating my bloodstream, leaving boils on my skin, dark rings around my eyes, and strange dark matter around my teeth.

It would have killed me, of course, and the police would have thought it was a drug overdose, or a mysterious stroke—provided, of course, that they weren't in on it, too. I realised what was happening when Smithy began telling me how awful I looked that day. By 'telling me', I mean he followed me around the house yelling it at me. We were in Smithy's meth house: a bright, brand new, three-bedroom house—rented by Smithy from a large corporation that owned every second house in the neighbourhood—in Pakenham, 61 kilometres south-east of Melbourne, in a little pocket of new housing in a little valley surrounded by bushland and farms. Pakenham is right on the tip of the Gippsland/Latrobe Valley region, and is considered to be one of the most badly affected meth areas in Australia.

It began when I rejected Smithy's sexual advances. He went on the offensive: 'What do you think *you* look like from the outside?'

*Oh dear*, I thought.

'You look revolting,' he said, a packed bong in his hand, lighter flicking on and off. 'And the way you smell, Jesus—people have been commenting, it's rank—the whole end of the house stinks because of your bedroom.'

*Oh dear*.

I took a sniff of myself and, yes, it would seem I smelt a bit off—something had been seeping out of my veins in an unseemly, abject manner. Never one to be distracted from the task, I asked, 'Can I have that bong if you're not going to smoke it?'

'No!' he growled, the refusal seeming to shoot out of his nose.

Each room of the house provoked a new criticism: the unused vegetables in the fridge revealed I wasn't eating properly; the dry, unclean bathroom revealed I wasn't showering, while the bathroom cabinet revealed I wasn't using deodorant; the bong bowl in the bedroom was a clear indicator I had been smoking too many of his cones.

'Go on, go and look at ya self in the bloody mirror.'

I walked to the mirror in his bedroom—the light was switched off, and only a little bit of light crept in through the bottom of the closed curtains.

I looked at my reflection, and saw a very attractive person with glowing skin, so I walked back out of the room and told Smithy, 'I look hot, as always.'

'I think you should have a closer look,' he mumbled. 'Why don't you go and have a look at your teeth if you think you look so good, you fucking pea-brain.'

This time, as I stared in the mirror, I saw poison oozing out of my skin, pus-y pimples, dark rings around my eyes, strange blisters on my neck, and blackened teeth. What *was* going on?

I mean, really—there was something *really* messed-up going on. I started to think that perhaps Smithy wasn't being nasty with his attack—perhaps he was trying to tell me something. My previous understanding of reality as more or less safe, fairly predictable—though at times somewhat mysterious and ambiguous—began to rupture from beneath those bathroom tiles. It might have been some kind of ontological earthquake right there in Pakenham, only the break wasn't so much a big crack as an all-encompassing clear line of revelation: Smithy's outburst, the dark rings around my eyes, why my ex had left me years ago and why he now looked so feminine, why our other roommate sometimes looked at me strangely, why my friend Beck had stopped talking to me a few weeks ago, why Smithy kept telling me to look in the mirror, my sunken cheeks, why my parents hadn't called me for the past few weeks, and why I had those strange blisters. Finally a light of revelation had begun to flash: *everyone is trying to kill me.* My parents had organised it, my friends were carrying it out, and I was dying—slowly, silently—without a single ally, and with poison seeping out of every pore.

So now to the point at which I rang my dad—my gentle, generous, non-offensive dad—to reveal what I had finally figured out. Dad answered the phone half-asleep.

'G'day, mate.'

'Don't try to pretend everything is normal, Dad! I've worked out what's going on—please don't do this to me. You have to understand, Dad, I was only joking in that story about killing you and Mum, it was only a story, and it wasn't even about you, and now I know what is going on—', and on I went, talking a mile a minute. I told him about the crystal meth, the arsenic, the secret sex-change, the animal-liberationist plot, the money exchanged with Smithy's seedy drug-dealer friends, until finally

Dad said the inevitable, 'Um, mate, I think I might put you on to your mum.'

But I hung up the phone and walked into the lounge room — where Smithy was now entertaining a couple of seedy-looking guests — saying, 'I know what's going on, you rats …'

They started laughing. 'Oh fuck, you're a tripper, Luke,' one said. 'Never a dull moment when you're around.'

'You writing one of your stories again, Luke?' Smithy asked, smiling.

I had been telling tall tales back then. Some of them took on a life of their own; in some I killed everybody I knew in graphic detail, often in the most unlikely ways, and with the most unlikely accomplices. These fantasies often took place in a post-apocalyptic world with no police, and where the council served only to take the bodies away.

Confused, I rang my parents back. My mum answered, and when she asked why I thought that they were trying to kill me, I realised there were a few gaps in my logic; that, in fact, I had been deeply mistaken. Beyond my imagination, there were memories which revisited me like movies: I started sweating as teenagers dressed in bright-red uniforms called me a faggot; then I was in Year 9 and my best friend was throwing my pencil case on the ground and telling me to sit somewhere else; then I was homeless and stealing food. Soon I was in tears, talking about the bullying I'd gone through in high school, and what had happened since, in a conversation that lasted nearly six hours.

For many chronic users, self-deception can become extreme paranoia, and sometimes full-blown psychosis. And at some stage in the preceding weeks, I had slipped into meth addiction. Why did I look like that? Because I'd been on a meth bender for a couple of weeks, and had completely forgotten to brush my teeth. What had actually happened? I had been using the drug for nearly two months, and I'd become an addict. I'd used it bit by bit, here and there. I'd feel so tired I'd take a bit more, until my mind got so twisted I lost track of how much I was actually using, and how much my behaviour had changed. I had become what I later realised was one of the estimated 100,000 Australians addicted to crystal meth.

On this particular afternoon, Smithy—the junkie and jailbird—had started that conversation because he was either worried about me, or he was experiencing some kind of psychosis himself. And yes, it took *this* person to tell me that what I needed to do was settle down and go to bed—but, before that, I really, really needed to use some Listerine.

I knew long before I moved in that Smithy dealt drugs from his house, and that meth use and meth users were near-constant companions. There were always people coming and going, with plenty of 'drug dramas'—fights, conspiracies, drug dealers arguing—that generally arose during the comedown of the meth cycle, and then vanished once the drug wore off. People from the local boarding house often used Smithy's place to shoot-up in. Many of Smithy's friends were also thieves, who robbed display homes to help support themselves and their habits. They would sneak out in the early hours of the morning, coming back with fridges, washing machines, or microwaves that they would then trade for drugs.

In short, Smithy seemed like the right subject for a story. So I came up with the idea of moving in with him to tell the ultimate story of meth addiction. Fresh out of a mind-numbing business-law job (I had retired from journalism to become a lawyer, but that didn't quite work out, and I never finished the qualification), I told Smithy about my idea, and he agreed to participate. ('As long as you pay your bloody rent, I don't care what you bloody do.') So I rented a room for $130 a week. What could possibly go wrong?

As it turned out, I got addicted to meth while living in a house to write a story about a meth dealer and his drug-addict mates. I cooked my brain so badly on meth that, after a few months, I genuinely lost track of the fact I was writing a story; I stopped taking notes, and became fixated on a series of non-existent events, with myself at the centre. So, yes—as you may have gathered—I got a story, a very good story. Only it wasn't the one I was expecting: I didn't bank on becoming a psychotic meth addict myself. I spent virtually the entirety of Melbourne's beautiful autumn inside that house, gradually losing my mind. Slowly and unwittingly, over three months, I became an addict—replete with meth sores, violent outbursts, an obscenely bloody needle-stick injury, and shamefully long, disgustingly sweaty masturbation marathons. I met and had to make a few mad escapes from some very shady characters. I became embroiled in small-time crime, pointless, never-ending loopy conversations, and never-ending, taboo-busting sexual fantasies (Smithy's and my own).

I became violent and threatening, particularly toward my parents; in one particularly memorable phone message I left for my tattooed, retired-slaughterman father, I put on my best ABC-news voice to explain that I would come up to Queensland and 'kill you with my bare fucking hands'. Grandiosity, bloodlust, bad memories, and paranoia can be a rather unsavoury combination. In short, I went from being nice, respectable Luke to being 'an ugly, sweaty, desperate animal' in scenes vaguely reminiscent of the promo for the 1971 classic Australian film *Wake in Fright*.

June 2015: It was a winter's night in Nowra, a stunning farm-and-bush town surrounded by mountains 160 kilometres south of Sydney. Inside the Bomaderry RSL club's conference room, 100-odd people watched on as Tracey Reece told her story through a microphone.

'He told us that there were people (probably adults) coming to the back gate of the school, and when we approached the school they said that it wasn't possible, that they had teachers on duty down there,' she said. Reece, a woman in her early forties with short, bleached hair, began to quiver.

'Later on, a year down the track, we got told by our son that was where he was originally given it and asked to sell it,' she explained to the police-sponsored Shoalhaven community forum on ice. Reece was talking about her son, now seventeen, who had been fifteen when he encountered meth, reportedly buying it from a dealer at the gates of his high school.

'He went from being this beautiful little innocent boy who couldn't lie to his mum, to [being] very angry. He turned into a monster,' Reece said, tears streaming down her cheeks, as a slight murmur of agreement started to buzz around the room.

When a person becomes a meth addict, they change. 'Monster' is a common and often appropriate noun used to describe what they have become. The word derives from the Latin *monstrum*, which means an aberrant occurrence, usually a sign that there is something wrong with the natural order. Over time, monsters appeared in mythology as sub-human beasts, as nasty, bloodthirsty, amoral, and ugly as they were large.

Our long-running fear of monsters shows how the terror and sadness often experienced by those close to a meth addict, particularly as they begin to fall, is of a profound, archetypal, and very understandable variety; yet it is also one that is open to interpretation. We know the story of Robert Louis Stevenson's 1886 classic, *The Strange Case of Dr Jekyll and Mr Hyde*. Dr Henry Jekyll takes an experimental new potion with the hope it will help his ill father — only to be transformed into the smaller, uglier Edward Hyde, who then kills two innocent people. Dr Jekyll vows never to turn into Mr Hyde again, but the transformations increase in frequency and do not, eventually, even require the potion to take effect. Dr Jekyll's ability to turn back into himself diminishes, and ultimately Mr Hyde takes over; Dr Jekyll never returns. We never really know to what extent Mr Hyde was simply Dr Jekyll's socially repressed dark side.

People do strange and often terrible things when they meet the beast within. We never hear the story from Mr Hyde's point of view, though in the beginning, at least, Dr Jekyll has a full memory of what Mr Hyde did. We are left with the question of how much agency Dr Jekyll really had, and this in turn makes me ask myself some uncomfortable questions about what I got out of living on meth.

Leading up to my own addiction, I had observed this strange transformative process in many of the people closest to me, and I was often as upset as I was confused and alienated by the changes they went through on the way to becoming meth-heads. Before crystal meth started making it big in the news in late 2013, I had seen a key collection of my friends sliding into addiction, from 2011 onward. This included my cousin, my ex-boyfriend, my old friend Beck, and her ex-partner, Smithy, who—despite two restraining orders that forbade them from seeing each other—lived just around the corner from her, and visited regularly.

Most had lost his or her job, as well as any sense of ordinary meaning and direction in life. They had become loose with the truth, although at times it wasn't clear if they were being manipulative, or if they believed their own lies, or a combination of the two. Their lives seemed to revolve around the drug, but they had either limited insight into this fact, or a kind of 'fuck you, sheep' response to the conventional idea that life was better when you were not using drugs. A few had lost teeth. A few had turned to crime; for instance, when my cousin discovered meth at the age of thirty-seven, he went from being a sulky, reclusive pot-smoker with a job and a mortgage to being an unemployed burglar who'd stolen from his mum, and was living in a car in a public park. Dinner—on the rare occasions he felt like eating—was sausages cooked on the park BBQ. Perhaps this doesn't seem all that bad when you're high on meth. Perhaps he found that lifestyle more exciting, more dramatic, more relaxing, even, than having a mortgage and an alarm clock to worry about. In any event, it was a phenomenon that begged serious questions, and I wanted to find out what the allure of this drug was—what it was providing that users' everyday lives weren't.

I had taken meth before, and enjoyed it, but I didn't think it warranted throwing your life away. What's more, the meth addicts I knew had taken just about every other kind of drug, and still managed to be semi-functional, crime-free, and predominantly sane—so why couldn't these users manage their meth in the way they had managed their use of other drugs? And hadn't the issue already been and gone? We had already heard about meth in the mid-2000s. What had changed by the time meth began to attract more and more of the public's attention in 2013? Was this just an old issue being re-hashed?

Actually, no—I would learn that this increased attention coincided with a purer version of the drug flooding Australia's drug markets. The first real indication that this purer form of methamphetamine—crystallised meth or 'ice' (as opposed to the powdered variety that we had heard so much about in the 2000s)—had made its way to our shores came in around 2011, when drug experts around the country started getting phone calls from health workers on the ground in Nowra, south of Sydney, saying that crystallised meth was being widely abused, and wreaking havoc, in its Aboriginal communities.

For reasons that are still not completely clear, however, it would be Victoria, and particularly regional Victoria, that would be saturated by ice. And it began to be felt in extraordinarily horrific ways.

—

In the early hours of Friday 15 June 2012, 19-year-old Harley Hicks, a troubled young man who been separated from his parents at an early age and had a significant criminal record, was prowling around the dark, empty, eucalypt-lined streets of Long Gully, a suburb of Bendigo in central Victoria. On this cold winter morning, he had already robbed several houses, and wanted to find just one more before the sun broke. He was energised from smoking crystal meth when he entered the old Victorian-style house in Eaglehawk Road. He was carrying a shoulder bag, and a makeshift baton crafted from copper wire and electrical tape. He first found a wallet on the kitchen bench that contained thousands of dollars set aside by the tenants, Matthew Tisell and Casey Veal—people Hicks vaguely knew—for a bond to move into a new house the next night.

He grabbed whatever he could find—a set of scales, and a pair of sunglasses. Then he made his way to the front of the house, where he searched two rooms before entering the bedroom of 10-month-old Zayden Veal, who was sleeping with a baby monitor next to him. With neither a motive nor a feeling of any particular ill will towards Zeal's parents, Hicks unplugged the baby monitor, and then hit Zayden repeatedly with his homemade baton in the face and torso. After several blows, the baby slipped into permanent darkness; the subsequent post-mortem revealed that Zayden had sustained horrific injuries to his face and scalp, the pathologist noting that Zayden had been hit not only with the length of the baton, but also with the end of it, from which copper wire protruded.

In total, Zayden was found to have received at least 25 injuries to the face, and a minimum of eight injuries to the scalp. Hicks pleaded not guilty. The jury disagreed, and Justice Stephen Kaye sentenced the teenaged baby-killer to thirty-two years in prison before he would have the prospect of parole, telling Hicks before sentencing him that there was not 'even the slightest indication by you of any pity or sympathy for the baby, whose life you had taken, or for his family, whose lives you have shattered. Rather, you seemed totally oblivious and impervious to such human feelings'.

This new drug, crystal meth—created in Japan nearly a century ago, originally available over the counter at pharmacies, and then made popular by American bikie gangs after it was made illegal—was enjoyed so much by Australia's drug-using population that many users quickly became addicts, and others found their lives spiralling quickly out of control.

In early 2013, a joint state-federal police operation made a discovery that shocked them deeply. The investigation, which involved the Australian Federal Police (AFP), customs officials, New South Wales Police, and the Australian Crime Commission (ACC), was prompted by a tip-off from a member of the public about suspicious activity at a storage facility in West Ryde, Sydney. After monitoring the facility's comings and goings for some time, the police intercepted three large containers, supposedly full of cleaning chemicals, which had been shipped from southern China. The raid turned up an astonishing 585 kilograms of high-quality crystal meth, with an estimated street value of $430 million. As a sign of things to come, the three men arrested were from different territories who had been working together to traffic the drug—a Singaporean, an Australian, and a Hong Kong man. Reporting on the bust, among many others, was the BBC, and *The Huffington Post*, which noted that 'Australia seems to be a popular destination for drug smugglers'.

The 2013 Australian Crime Commission Illicit Drug Data Report (which was released in April 2014) indicated that this 585-kilogram haul was just the tip of the … well, iceberg.

According to the report, the weight of amphetamines-group detections by customs increased by 516 per cent from 347.3 kilograms in 2011–12 to 2138.5 kilograms in 2012–13. Nationally, the number of amphetamines seizures increased by 39 per cent from 15,191 in 2011–12 to 21,056 in 2012–13. Unsurprisingly, the problem began to be noticed at rehabs, hospitals, police stations, and medical centres around the nation, as many drug users quickly moved to more regular use of this high-potency amphetamine. While the media was actually slow to recognise this new trend at first, there is no doubt it was making an impact on the community. It just took a little while for the problem to make news.

Jazmin-Jean Ajbschitz was a small, dark 18-year-old from the inner-Sydney suburb of Ultimo. When she was killed in mid-2011, the coroner who examined her corpse noted that the injuries to her ribs were so severe—her heart had been partially torn—that they were typical of injuries seen in victims of high-speed car crashes. Jazmin-Jean, however, had been killed by her boyfriend—who was high on crystal meth at the time—because she had ended her relationship with him via a text message. Twenty-seven years old at the time of the murder, Sean Lee King was sentenced to twenty-five and a half years in prison in June 2013, saying he 'feels the pain every day' of knowing he murdered his ex-girlfriend.

More murders would follow, and although it was unclear just how much of a role the drug had played when the murderer had been on crystal meth, the killings often showed similar characteristics: they were senseless, often depraved, often perverted, recklessly violent, and often playfully sadistic.

About two months after King's sentencing, the then acting assistant commissioner, Doug Fryer, of the Victoria Police Intelligence and Covert Support Command, told the *Herald*

*Sun*: 'This is our new heroin.' Journalist Mark Dunn reported that in at least 12 murders committed or tried by courts over the preceding two years, crystal methamphetamine had been either used by the killer or was otherwise a suspected factor in the crime. Four of those killings involved young women—including two in Smithy's home suburb of Pakenham, in which both young women were senselessly killed in their homes—and others involved seemingly normal home robberies that became irrational, bloody, sadistic killings. So while it is true that murders occur all the time in Australia *without* the influence of crystal meth, police were beginning to see a clear pattern between certain types of homicides and the drug.

Around the same time I was living in the house, the Victorian parliament was running its inquiry into methamphetamine use—the Inquiry into the Supply and Use of Methamphetamines, Particularly Ice, in Victoria—with a final report to be delivered in August 2014. The report would receive 81 submissions, and conduct hearings all over the state. The committee would hear that nearly all drug rehabs had experienced an increase in the number of clients citing methamphetamine as their problem drug, often leading to six-week-or-longer waiting lists at many publicly funded facilities. Even getting to see a drug counsellor on the public purse could involve 10-day-plus waits, which was time enough for someone to relapse and not have the presence of mind to turn up to their next appointment.

Parliamentary submissions indicated that general psychologists and health practitioners lacked the expertise to deal with meth addiction, with conventional therapies such as cognitive behavioural therapy often found to have limited utility in treating a condition that wears down a person's reasoning and risk-assessment skills. Meanwhile, meth addicts and drug users more generally often complained about feeling stigmatised by health professionals, and having a deep sense of shame in accessing treatment for a behaviour which centres around an illicit substance.

In Victoria's parliamentary inquiry, frontline community workers gave evidence that at times was quite shocking. Anex, a group that works principally as a needle exchange for drug users, wrote in their submission:

> Casual users quickly progress to harmful use ... long-term adverse effects of the consumption of methamphetamine are well documented and include dependence, cardiovascular complications, neurotoxic effects associated with the development of psychomotor disturbances similar to Parkinson's disease, and psychosis.

Dr Mathew Frei, of the Turning Point Alcohol and Drug Centre, told the Victorian parliamentary inquiry:

> Sometimes we see people getting very overheated, and rhabdomyolysis is a breakdown of muscles which can lead to kidney failure. These are relatively rare but very significant toxic effects of methamphetamine. Occasionally we see cardiac events. You can imagine that a drug that increases your heart rate and increases your blood pressure might bring risk of a cardiac event, like heart failure or a heart attack, and occasionally we have seen seizures and actual strokes—so, injuries to the brain.

Melbourne City Mission reported that homeless meth-using clients 'typically present to the service paranoid and aggressive—they can often be violent and threatening and display poor emotional self-regulation—including a reduced capacity or willingness to take responsibility for actions'.

It was obvious from the inquiry that regional Victoria was badly affected, though it was not clear whether this was because there were simply more users and abusers, or because treatment services were not as readily available. The Victorian Aboriginal Legal Aid Service told the committee that there was an 'ice epidemic' occurring in the Sunraysia area:

> We have had about seven suicides due to the use of ICE this year alone. … We have also seen an increase in Hume, Echuca, and Bendigo … At a statewide level estimates of the percentage of clients using ICE at the time of offending vary from around 15 per cent to 60 per cent.

In October 2014, *The Sydney Morning Herald* would report:

> Amphetamine use, particularly crystal methamphetamine or 'ice', has risen by up to 180 per cent over two years in some regional centres like Coffs Harbour, Cessnock, and Wagga Wagga. But the scourge is also infiltrating smaller towns — such as Moree, Broken Hill, and Casino — that had never heard of the cheap and destructive drug 10 years ago.

Over the 2014–15 period, an alleged Queensland Rebels gang member would be charged with giving a 2-year-old boy the drug ice; Harriet Wran — the youngest daughter of former New South Wales premier Neville Wran — was found sleeping rough and using ice in the lead up to being charged with murder; industrial-scale meth labs were being found in the ACT; a group of young fallen sports stars started a multi-million dollar ice syndicate in Wangaratta complete with written instructions when a new member joined; a *Four Corners* program would broadcast allegations that bikie gangs were getting people addicted to ice as young as thirteen so the victim would manufacture and sell the drug for them; dozens of babies would be born around the nation addicted to meth; a 20-year-old in Melbourne's south-eastern suburbs would rack up 107 charges on a three-month ice-fuelled crime spree; and a paraplegic West Australian man known as 'Hot Wheels' would be charged and convicted with dealing meth, which he kept hidden in his wheelchair. A UNSW report published in June 2015 indicates that in 2011 there were 101 methamphetamine-related deaths in Australia, up from 85 in 2010. Preliminary projections they made for 2012 and 2013 of up to 170 deaths suggest a continuing rising trend.

Australia is just one nation among many grappling with this strange, dream-like drug. To be more precise, the reason we have high-purity crystal meth in Australia is because worldwide production of the drug has gone into overdrive over the past five years.

Throughout western civilisation, monsters, such as Medusa, have long been associated with something dangerously alluring—at times, people can't help but engage with a monster, even if they know there are terrible consequences of doing so. Other monsters lure victims with enchanting music, drawing the unwary in, and leaving nothing but dead bones and rotting flesh all around them.

Being told that you are behaving like a monster when you're on ice feels completely at odds with the way you *actually* feel when you are on the drug. And the way you feel is totally different to the way you look; a reminder that drugs don't become addictive because they make you feel as if you're eating razor blades—they become addictive because they feel bloody awesome. Meth feels … spectacular. It's cheap, it lasts for a long time, and when you first start using it, you get a lot of work done—all while having the time of your life. What could be better than that?

People take drugs for a number of different reasons: because they are happy, as well as because they are sad; to celebrate, as well as to escape. People often take meth to lose weight, or to share an experience with friends; they take it to let go, and also to enhance life. And when they take it, there is nothing to suggest that evil or suffering might be just around the corner. To further complicate matters, there is no single agreed approach on what works for treating addiction. There are also a lot of different theories about what causes addiction in the first place—genetic theory, moral theory, disease theory, learning and behavioural theory, socio-cultural theory. Our culture, too, sends mixed messages about drug-taking that make it seem at once a moral failing, and somewhat glamorous. Despite being an age-old problem, the drug addict that exists today is a perfect metaphor for a consumer culture with an insatiable pit of desire, and a tendency to have us want things we don't really need.

But more so, there is something about the particular character of a meth high and meth addiction that mirrors the style of our culture. A dose of meth makes you feel as if you have won an award, been offered sex by a very attractive person, and are taking off in an aeroplane—all at the same time. You feel warm, calm, coherent, and crystal-clear; meth inflames your ego, your libido, and your sense of being comfortable with danger. You feel confident to the point of feeling superior—every memory of your achievements, every compliment you have ever received, seems to rush to your consciousness simultaneously. Indeed, it's hard *not* to think you are amazing if you can feel so successful just by putting a needle in your arm. You feel fulfilled, purposeful, and excited. You also feel seedy, admittedly, but in a cool, edgy way. For the most part, we had loads of fun in Smithy's house; we sat up and talked all night, we had crazy conversations and laughed so much we gave ourselves stitches. There is often an intimacy in drug circles that can be hard to find in other parts of society.

Crystal meth, and the wonderfully mysterious vortex it plunges its users into, can make you feel that your life is one big, magical, lucid dream where anything is possible, everything and everyone revolves around you, and consequences are not binding. But then there is the flip side, when the magic potion wears off, and the dreams become nightmares. Crystal meth is a bit like the 'old religion' spells in the TV show *Merlin*—you end up feeling as if nature is punishing you for messing with the equilibrium.

Meth, at its heights, fulfils the gap between what American sociologist Daniel Bell describes as 'The Cultural Contradictions of Capitalism': the contradiction between the cultural sphere of consumerist, instant self-gratification and hedonism, and the demand, in the economic sphere, for hard-working, productive individuals.

This also gives us a chance to reflect on drugs in western culture, the modern concepts of addiction, and problematic drug use. In their book *High culture: reflections on addiction and modernity*, American philosophy academics Anna Alexander and Mark S. Roberts write:

> Western Culture—the Bible and the heroic myths, Orphic cults and mysteries, as well as the history of testimonial writing—contains numerous references to these substances taken solely for the purpose of altering the mind. Their potential energy has conquered the earth, and established communication between various cultures and peoples … these substances have filtered pathways between people of different worlds from the tribal to the modern, and have, moreover, opened passages for us that have proved useful in a number of ways.

Along similar lines, others note that prohibition of drugs and the 'medicalisation of drug use' is a distinctly modern phenomenon. Australian academics David Moore and Suzanne Fraser analyse the work of American author Eve Sedgwick thus:

For Sedgwick, Western liberal societies reliance upon Enlightenment notions of autonomy, rationality and freedom have produced a central dualism: free will and compulsion. She argues that for as long as we have idealised and worshipped the idea of free will, we have also generated its opposite: the denigrated, devalued idea of compulsion. In this model we strive only for good: pure freedom. Dependence or reliance or compulsion to do anything becomes defined here as contamination and failure of the will.

Fraser and Moore also draw on the work of the French post-structuralist Jacques Derrida, who says that drugs are 'not a scientific concept' but a political category with norms usually tending on the side of the 'prohibitionist'. While it can be tempting to use our pre-existing gripes with 'society' to explain the widespread use of meth, there is an important caveat to this line of questioning. In his book *Methland: the death and life of an American small town*, which documents the drug culture of Oelwein, Iowa, Nick Reding suggests that meth use in the American mid-west can be understood, at least partially, within the context of the loss of traditional local industry to globalising forces, and the social and economic decline that followed. Yet history shows that meth use occurs across all sectors of society, and in times of both economic prosperity and social decline. In *Methamphetamine: its history, pharmacology, and treatment*, medical doctor and author Ralph Weisheit says that:

> drug surges can ignite quickly in conditions characterized by high availability, the absence of legal drug controls, a vulnerable population of users, and social and economic distress resulting from conditions such as cultural demoralization, mass unemployment, poverty, or mass migration. They may also arise in conditions of sudden economic prosperity, excess income, and

the search for new symbols of status and pleasure—conditions that spawned American amphetamine use after the Second World War and the cocaine surges of the 1980s.

With all that in mind, I think it's noteworthy that meth often leaves the user highly individualised, robot-like, and egotistical. It is a drug developed and spread in an age of technology, productivity, prohibition, a globalised economy, and the subsequent global black market that grew alongside it, and in a culture dominated by big pharmaceutical companies and a highly medicalised society.

My experience is not everyone's experience with the drug, and this is not necessarily how everybody becomes addicted. I have known many users over the years who use, even weekly, and still hold down jobs, and don't appear to be adversely affected.

I have had drug addictions before. I took time off from my job at triple j to spend two months in rehab in 2008; after breaking up with my partner and failing at a big work project, I used every drug I could lay my hands on—including heroin and powdered meth—until I was a blubbering, teary mess. But since leaving rehab, though I did crave meth from time to time, I had been able to stop myself using it many times. I believed my life was so full, and my addiction-strategies so sharpened, that I could live in the Pakenham house, take the drug occasionally, and still function well enough to write a profile piece about a chronic drug addict. In truth, however, and as I shall explain, there are complex reasons why I succumbed to the drug, which go beyond the fact that I was taking, and indeed injecting, a far stronger dose than I was used to. I had suffered trauma as a teenager, but addiction itself is complex: seventeen years of using drugs, regardless of my initial reasons for taking them, have created a void—a drug-shaped hole—in my heart that not only leaves me susceptible to the 'substance of the day', at times and to this day, but that still seems impossible to fill with something else. I have always preferred fantasy to reality—particularly fantasy of the self-aggrandising type. I am often irresponsible, reckless, volatile, self-involved. I hate rules and limitations, such as the fact that humans don't live forever, don't have wings and can't fly, and I can't deny that a syringe full of meth brings me pretty close to flying and feeling immortal. This book is partly an invitation for you to go on a journey with me as I try to identity and then exorcise, or at least mitigate, the problems in my own character that led me to addiction.

# Chapter Two

# Panic!

I GREW UP in a small, hilly, damp, conservative town called Emerald and I went to school in Pakenham, where Smithy's house is, and where much of this story takes place. I moved back to 'Packy' when I was twenty-eight, and I moved back again at thirty-four to write this book. How would I describe the place? Well, I quite like it; it's close to nature, but just an hour's train ride to the city. What does it look like? Well, it's ... pretty. It's a reasonably affluent working-class town, the last stop on the suburban train line, with mixed terrain and a mixture of people. It's not for everyone; one local suggested it's 'a place for fuckwits who can't afford to live anywhere else'. All personal taste aside, it's essentially a flatland, surrounded on its northern side by mile upon mile of damp, tough, mossy, fern-covered mountains.

In fact, two hundred years ago the Pakenham district was a marshy, fertile hunting ground for indigenous tribes, full of eels, and roos, and wallabies that would come down from the mountains to drink from the seemingly endless puzzle of lakes and swamplands. When the first white settlers arrived in the 1830s, they found nothing much but copperhead snakes, impenetrable bushland, swampy fields, and holes in the ground that were full of nasty, stinging bull ants.

The first commercial enterprise in town was a pub run by the original landowners, which was fittingly placed along what is now a major highway, then little more than a goat track, in an area of Pakenham called the Toomuc Valley. Eventually, more bushland would be cleared, and the kangaroos would leave and be replaced by acres of pig farms and quarries. In years to come, Pakenham—named after a British war general—was far enough away from 'civilisation' to attract a steady mix of anti-establishment entrepreneurs, rebels, misfits, working-class individualists, murderers, and people who wanted to live by their own rules.

The most dramatic event in the town's history—the 1879 Sly Grog Riot—seems perfectly fitting when considered today, as Pakenham had a significant number of home-brewers who made their living selling grog to the inhabitants of the shanty town that sat on the small rise in the middle of town. In March 1879, the police turned up with a plan to seize the illicit spirits, only to be confronted by a hundred-strong mob armed with pick handles, sticks, and anything else they could find. The police retreated, and decided to simply ignore the illegal grog trade from then onwards.

For a long time, Pakenham had a reputation as a bogan farm-town. In the last fifteen years, however, its open grasslands have been filled with monotonous, homogenised, terracotta-roofed housing with multiple living areas and tiny backyards. Between 2007 and 2012, the suburb's population grew from 20,000 to 34,000. The towns surrounding Pakenham also grew quickly, and in the last five years Pakenham has become connected to part of the mass suburbia of south-east Melbourne.

Today, a single creek runs through town, creating a dividing line between new Pakenham's sparkling suburban areas, which have their own wetlands and cultural centre, and old Pakenham's simple, nostalgic, even earthy mix of old farmhouses, commission houses, crab apple trees, 1980s rentals, and big, beautiful white gums.

One of the last areas to be eaten up was the Toomuc Valley, which had remained a farmland for around a hundred and fifty years until it was sold to a massive corporate property developer in 2010. Now a residential village tucked away from the rest of Pakenham, the valley is still surrounded by beautiful hills that are covered in a combination of virgin bush and hobby farms. Most of the hills are so steep that it takes a very fit person (or, in my case, a highly psychotic meth-flushed person, contemplating how he was going to counter a murderous plot or expose a sadistic paedophile ring) to climb them. But if you did manage to climb to the top of one of them, you would see Pakenham's latest housing development. From a distance, the suburban outpost looks like a 1990s Sim City village with just enough parks to stop the locals from rioting. This is new Pakenham with a distinctive old Pakenham flavour: a mixture of rental properties and mortgaged houses, occupied by tradesmen, child-care workers, labourers, and the odd drug dealer. The little village is pleasant to look at, though if you look over the valley with a critical eye you will notice there is no community centre, oval, or anything that might resemble a means for people to run around or get together.

If you had been on one of the hills as the sun rose across the flatlands one Tuesday morning in the early autumn of 2014, you would have seen a half-moon lingering in the sky over the valley containing 30-or-so houses. If you had looked at one particular house, you might have seen that all the lights were on. Inside, sitting on his bed, was 42-year-old Rob Smith (Smithy), holding a syringe full of promise against the light cast by his bedroom lamp. An unskilled labourer in his everyday life, with needles the tools of his trade, he flicked the syringe with care and precision. Pouring white crystals from a clear, plastic sachet bag into a tablespoon full of boiling water, he mixed it with the end of the syringe, which he then used to crush the crystals until they became a white liquid. He tore off part of a cigarette and placed it in the mixture, took the lid off the fit, put the needle into the mixture, and drew it into the needle. He was a figure of concentration and purpose: efficient, careful, and productive.

I was also in that house, asleep. Beck, Smithy's ex-girlfriend, and near-permanent houseguest, was waiting outside my door, having had a shot of meth not long before. The buzz had sent her first into a talking spin, and then to the hallway cupboard, where she pulled out the vacuum cleaner and began vacuuming all the floors enthusiastically, a thin trail of blood dripping from her arm. Beck was letting me — her best friend of nearly twenty years — sleep for an extra hour before delivering the good news: Smithy had decided to give me tick.

I had been living in the house for three weeks at this stage, and I'd had just one shot of meth so far — due to both my desire to keep my usage irregular and to my lack of money.

She woke me with a couple of taps, saying: 'I told Smithy you were avoiding going over there because you owed him money and felt guilty taking more of his drugs. So he's happy to shout you until you get paid.'

'Okay, that's really nice. Thanks, mate,' I said, not wanting to give away that I'd hoped that by *not* asking for tick, Smithy would eventually get so horny and off-his-face that he'd offer me some anyway. I also didn't want to give away how excited I was about taking the drug. After all, I was there on assignment — work wasn't supposed to be so much fun.

I walked into the bedroom to see Smithy putting the finishing touches on my shot.

'Packin' 'em in Pakenham,' he said.

I rolled my eyes at his failed attempt at humour, and thanked him for the tick. He was ready to inject me, so I pumped up my arm and smacked the underside of my elbow to make a vein visible.

As the syringe was brought forward, I felt as if I was waiting for a Christmas present. Not every meth trip is the same, though they are almost always good if you don't do it all the time — even then, the effect of a syringe full of meth will always be better than doing your taxes, or working out how much of your pay will go on your rent. On this morning, my mouth watered, my throat tickled, and I took a deep breath in anticipation. He slipped the needle in painlessly; as it hit the vein, the syringe filled with deep, red blood — signifying that an exciting taboo had been broken.

As I later learned, when crystal meth enters the brain, it affects those neurons that contain dopamine, a feel-good chemical. On this day, the meth travelled up the blood in my arm, and was quickly absorbed into my brain's grey matter, going directly to its reward centre. My brain was flushed with dopamine; at the same time, my serotonin levels increased, improving my mood, while my noradrenaline levels dropped, drastically reducing my feeling of stress and anxiety. Until I took meth, I didn't believe it was possible for a human to feel so relaxed, alert, confident, euphoric, calm, and energised at the same time. I felt love, sex, danger, and mystery, right through my skin, all over my skin, enlarging my heart to the size of a balloon as I floated off into a land of dream and dance and immortality, excited by my rejection of everything I'd been taught about hard work being the only thing that can bring real happiness. With morning light just starting to seep through the bottom of the closed curtains, I put the stereo on in the lounge room and danced like a muppet. I felt energised by an edgy feeling of superiority, as if all the stupid, ordinary straights getting up for work were being 'left behind'.

The rest of the day went pretty much the same way (full of rampant stupidity), and is difficult to piece together as a coherent story. So let me explain it as best I can:

- Beck asked everyone who entered the house that day whether they liked penises, but so softly that none of them could hear her.
- Smithy asked me at least a dozen times whether Beck had been sneaking off at night to have sex with men in the bushes.
- A large refrigerator-repair man visiting from Kalgoorlie tried to convince me of a secret UN plan called 'Agenda 21' to reduce the world's population to less than 500,000.
- Beck spent approximately six hours playing *Zombie Apocalypse* on her iPad.

But—as they say—'it was all just a dream'. All good things must come to an end, everything that goes up must come down, and so on. Eventually, the balloon ran out of its proverbial helium, and I slowly floated back to earth. Before a big meth crash, you often find yourself on just the right level—not too up and not too down, the perfect time to get back to work. I was, after all, living in that house to find out how my friends had become hooked on meth (and, no, in retrospect, the irony of asking this after having such an outrageous time on meth is not lost on me).

Later that day, Smithy was sitting on the edge of his bed, wearing an Adidas tracksuit and a look of concentrated fury, discussing his theories of what had gone on during New Year's Eve behind his back (which I shall explain shortly), and going to the mirror every now and then to squint, and rub his face. It seemed as good a time as any for me to raise the issue of meth addiction.

'So, Smithy, I guess what I wanted to ask you about is how you fell into meth in that two years or so I didn't see you?'

Smithy gave me a look of horror, followed by one of suspicion. 'Well, you used to just use a bit of truckie speed on the weekends, and smoke bongs during the week, and now you use meth all the time,' I continued. 'I'm just wondering how that happened.'

Smithy kept staring at me silently.

'Y'know, no judgement here, mate. I just want to know how you managed to get so into meth,' I said.

His suspicion turned to mild aggression: 'I don't fucking use it all the time—who told you that? You always listen to everyone else, you always take everybody else's side, you'll listen to what everyone else has to say before asking me whether it's true.'

'Well,' I said, slowly and carefully, like a dog-catcher cautiously approaching a pit-bull. 'It's kind of obvious—'

'How?'

I looked at Smithy with his blotchy skin, a confused expression on his face, and the swabs, two used syringes, and used spoons sitting on either side of him.

'I can tell you this, Smithy, because you're a good bloke and my friend, and I can be honest with you: your skin, the way you look, you've lost so much weight, you don't work anymore—'

'There's nothing wrong with the way I look,' he said, his face flushed with blood. 'All this boils down to is people talking about me. I knew it, I knew it, I had a feeling this was going on. Arseholes saying shit about me behind my back, spreading shit, saying I'm a fucking paedophile, Beck telling people not to visit me. Why does no fucking cunt visit me? Because people are fucking spreading shit, that's why. So next time someone says Smithy is a junkie, why not, rather than just accept it as gospel, come and ask me if it's true?'

'So are you?'

'Am I what?'

'Y'know, a junkie?'

'No!' he roars. 'It's fucking Beck. She's just trying to fucking cover for her own fuck-ups—'

'You mean cover for her own meth use?'

'No fuckwit — to cover-up for New Year's Eve,' he said. 'I suppose you're going to take her side about that as well?'

And so we moved on to the topic of New Year's Eve, when he was convinced Beck stole his acid, and had sex with one of his friends in the bushes.

Before I moved into the house, I had asked Beck about her meth use as well. Like Smithy, she would ask for evidence, and when I provided it she would dispute it. At other times, she wouldn't answer directly, but would instead put her hand on my knee and say something like, 'I know your heart's in the right place, mate.' Then she'd change the topic to something she knew would interest me, before I had the chance to realise that that was what she'd done.

Meth users are often highly paranoid, and genuinely lose track of the 'truth' somewhere along the way. In most circumstances, they wouldn't answer a trusted friend honestly about how much they were using, even if they *did* have the self-awareness to monitor it. And it's extremely difficult to keep track of meth use, as a user's perception of time speeds up at the same time as their reasoning skills slow down.

Beck and Smithy would not be the kind of people to answer government surveys — or, at least, not honestly — and nor did they ever get medical treatment for their addictions. I wonder how many other meth addicts answer phone surveys by saying they either don't use meth very much or perhaps not at all, while they are surrounded by their used needles, with tin foil wrapped around their heads. I know from my own experience that meth can eat away at your self-awareness — to put it mildly — so the idea that there are accurate national records about how many people use meth, how much meth is used, and the harm that arises from it, makes me deeply suspicious. And when I see how low the most respected survey, the government's National Drug Strategy Household Survey (NDSHS), shows meth use to be, my suspicions are heightened. Why? The NDSHS, which is carried out by the Australian Institute of Health and Welfare (AIHW), reports that the prevalence of methamphetamine use in Australia and Victoria has remained relatively stable since 2001. This puts meth use at around 2.5 per cent of the population.

This raises a critical question: why would the NDSHS indicate no increase in the number of people using meth, when we are all so convinced it is such a problem? Are their surveys unreliable? Or is it the case that we are in the grip of a moral panic over meth that's affecting a far smaller cohort than we assume, and that I, for instance, was always wrong to assume that, just because I had known people who were addicted and didn't want to admit it, this was a broad social problem?

Indeed, on the other side of the debate, there are those who suggest that there is no 'meth epidemic' — that meth is not a disease or virus-like problem that is spreading uncontrollably around the community. Some suggest that the sense of crisis we have about the drug is driven by a media beat-up, self-interested bureaucracies, health agencies trying to get more funding, and by politicians driving their own agendas. Professor David Moore, for example, says that the public conversation around methamphetamine tends to be simplistic, panic-driven, and hyperbolic, leading to the perception that methamphetamine use is more prevalent and dangerous than the evidence suggests it is.

Could it be that our collective understanding of the 'meth problem' is being driven by a panicked approach that fails to take into account individual responsibility and pre-existing human foibles? Or, conversely, is this perspective a kind of relativist, media-studies framework that waters down the reality that meth abuse causes genuine human suffering?

Moore and his co-author Robin Dwyer, in an article

published in the *International Journal of Drug Policy* in 2013, do not definitively answer this question, but they do argue that catastrophising messages not only stigmatise users and reduce their willingness to get treatment, but also that disproportionate attitudes may lead to hard-line, punitive legal approaches to drugs that will inevitably make the situation worse. The pair also suggest that:

> Policy and health promotion concerning methamphetamine should: (i) develop a less alarmist and more nuanced portrayal of the relationship between methamphetamine use and psychosis; (ii) avoid portraying psychosis (or hallucinations, visions and paranoia) as always and inevitably distressing and pathological — such messages are unlikely to resonate with consumers ... and (iii) avoid representing methamphetamine consumers as out-of-control, dangerous, threatening, and irrational.

Another viewpoint is that of Columbia University's charismatic, dreadlocked associate professor of psychiatry Carl Hart, who Moore cites as a significant influence on his work. 'Drug panics are a natural response to any threatening problem, but such panics are often exploited to advance the power, prestige, or financial interests of individuals and institutions claiming ownership of the problem,' Hart says.

Hart argues that it is moral panic and media hysteria that distorts the truth about meth, and not the attitudes of the users themselves. One of the most salient points about the meth phenomenon is that the 'vast majority of meth users are not addicted,' he says, and that when a drug user is doing poorly in life, drugs become the scapegoat. 'People stop looking for other reasons for problems once they know drugs are involved ... that way, you don't have to look at more complicated problems.'

Bearing all this in mind, there is nevertheless strong evidence about increasing meth use in Australia that is hard to repudiate. When we look at the health figures, and hear stories from people working on the front line, there is a lot of evidence to suggest that the meth problem is getting worse. Nationally, the number of amphetamine-related hospital admissions recorded in 2011–12 (2,895) was the highest since 1993–94 (which was, incidentally, the year that the first shipments of powdered methamphetamine arrived in Australia, as well as the year that ecstasy reached its peak popularity). What's more, these admissions had steadily increased over the previous three years. The figures from the health department are backed up not just by dozens of anecdotal reports by frontline workers, but by the crime statistics: the number of national arrests for all amphetamines (including ecstasy and speed) in Australia reached an all-time high of 22,189 over the 2012–13 period, which was a 32 per cent increase on the previous year. The number of clandestine laboratories detected nationally had more than doubled within a decade, increasing from 358 in 2003–04 to 757 in 2012–13. There was a 6.4 per cent decrease in the number of clandestine laboratories detected in Australia late in this period—from 809 in 2011–12 to 757 a year later—which was the first decrease since 2006–07. Despite this decrease, it was still the second-highest number of detections per year on record. Statistics and figures from state health departments also back the idea that the meth problem is ascending, as do the stories from rehab managers who say they now have a greater proportion of people seeking help because of methamphetamine.

So what's going on here? Are official government surveys failing to capture a group of transient, paranoid users who never seek help, lack the self-awareness to answer research groups properly, and lie about whether or not they are using meth (let alone whether or not it is causing them harm or psychosis)? Or are these surveys not even reaching the population group — such as the homeless, the mentally ill, and prisoners — who are statistically more likely to take meth?

This seems to be a controversial issue. The National Drug and Alcohol Research Centre (NDARC) declined to provide a person to be interviewed on whether the NDSHS figures were accurate, although a spokesperson conceded that their research doesn't cover homeless or imprisoned populations. Indeed, slightly different research cohorts might be part of the confusing impressions left in the media. An NDARC spokesperson, Lucy Burns, told *The Guardian* Australia that:

> The AIHW [the NDSHS] was a general population survey — which means they don't concentrate on people who might actually be in the drug market.

Perhaps, though, the answer is both simpler and more nuanced than it first seems. If you look more closely at the NDSHS data, you'll see that while meth use per capita isn't increasing, there has been a significant increase in the proportion of users taking it daily or weekly (from 9.3 per cent to 15.5 per cent), particularly among ice users (from 12.4 per cent to 25.3 per cent) between 2010 and 2013. What's more, it also shows that use of the less potent meth powder decreased significantly from 51 per cent to 29 per cent, while the use of ice (or crystal methamphetamine) more than doubled, from 22 per cent in 2010 to 50 per cent in 2013. From this, it can be concluded that while crystal meth is not taking over the community in 'pandemic proportions', many existing drug users — who once had hold of their drug use — are slipping into potentially addictive behaviour because a more potent drug is on the market. The fact that amphetamine users are using methamphetamine more often could also explain why there is more harm being caused. Crystal meth isn't 'recruiting' people with no drug history; instead, casual users of powdered meth — often referred to as 'speed' or just 'meth' — and ecstasy have found themselves taking a more powerful and far more addictive version of the class of drugs that they had thus far been able to use in moderation (although this may change as younger generations come through without prior experience of any other drugs, and find that crystal meth is available in the same way ecstasy or powdered meth had been for previous generations who eventually graduated to crystal-meth use). In this regard, we can say that while crystal meth is a significant social problem, there isn't really a 'meth epidemic' — at least not if we define 'epidemic' as a thing that spreads through the general community like an infectious disease — because it's pre-existing amphetamine users (not the population at large) who are being affected, albeit often very seriously.

In February 2016, NDARC released a report conducted by a research team that went beyond population surveys and instead measured data on treatment episodes for amphetamines, including people seeking counselling, rehabilitation, detoxification, and hospitalisation. The team, led by Professor Louisa Degenhardt, concluded that 'the number of regular methamphetamine users has almost tripled from 90,000 in 2009–2010 to 268,000 in 2013–2014'. Noting that their figures provided us with the first 'quantitative estimate of the scale of the problem of methamphetamine use in Australia', the study warned that methamphetamine dependence had more than doubled in people aged between fifteen and twenty-four between 2009–10 and 2013–14: 'Worryingly 1.14 per cent of young people aged 15–24 are estimated to be dependent on the drug compared with only 0.4 per cent in 2009–2010' the report, published in *The Medical Journal of Australia*, said.

ACC figures indicate that methamphetamine purity has risen, in Victoria, from approximately 20 per cent in the 2010–11 reporting period to more than 75 per cent in the 2012–13 period. In New South Wales, it rose over the same period from 9.5 per cent purity to 68 per cent; in Queensland, from 13 per cent to 52 per cent; in South Australia, from 31 per cent to 54 per cent; in West Australia, from 32 per cent to 50 per cent; and in Tasmania, from 9 per cent to 64 per cent.

Why is this purity rising? Over the last four years there has been far more methamphetamine coming into Australia from developing countries, particularly through the postal system via airmail. While we used to have powdered meth, the crystallised form is now far more common, and this form of the drug is far more potent (although, to confuse matters, they are both referred to as just 'meth' in street slang). Powdered meth and crystal meth are made the same way, with the same ingredients; it's just that 'crystallising' the 'base' involves a few more steps in the process.

The vast majority of the 500,000 Australians who used meth in the last twelve months are *not* dependent on it (though this does not necessarily mean that meth isn't having a negative impact on their lives). Dependence is a slippery concept in meth, but generally — if we accept that the official statistics are accurate — most meth users use occasionally, and most (although I remain suspicious of this self-reporting statistic, for reasons already stated) do not report harms such as psychosis, or commit crimes. Australia Bureau of Statistics drug-market modellers have calculated that there are approximately ten times more 'occasional' users of methamphetamine than there are 'heavy users'. This is not the case with heroin, where they estimate 'heavy users' outnumber 'occasional users'. Rebecca McKetin, a fellow at ANU's College of Medicine, Biology and Environment, estimates that there are around 100,000 addicts, or about 20 per cent of this number. ('Addict' refers to someone who is using more than once a week.)

In his presentation to the Victorian parliamentary committee on methamphetamine use, addiction specialist Dr David Jacka agreed, for the most part, that a combination of media reporting and a misunderstanding of the true nature of addiction has contributed to a perception that methamphetamine results in more serious dependency problems than is the case, at least compared to other drugs. Dr Jacka said:

> The vast majority of people never go beyond functional use. They never go beyond recreational use. It [meth] is nowhere near as addictive as cigarettes, nicotine ... Crack cocaine is a really good example of something that is much more addictive. Heroin is much more addictive. Methamphetamine, crack and ice are perhaps more addictive than ordinary amphetamines, but it is still of the order of 15 to 20 per cent of people who use the drug habitually will become dependent. It is not the majority by any means.

One of the key risks is that by focusing on the 'hard end' of drug use, we may miss opportunities to take a more preventative approach and address important but less severe issues among users. It is important not to accept without reservation accounts suggesting all users behave in a violent or psychotic manner, particularly after only occasional or short-term episodes of using the drug.

I do know one guy, a journalist, who says he uses meth every time he needs to move house, and finds the drug incredibly useful. I also know a woman who works as a drug counsellor who uses the drug just once a year—on New Year's Eve. Then there are the club bunnies—I've known many private-school kids who revel in the edginess of meth use, while still maintaining all the things that make them privileged. The meth use seemed to *enhance* their image; these were good-looking kids who loved extended after-parties, and saying things like, 'Oh no, a bit of three-thirty-itis' before smoking their crack pipe in the middle of the day. I've stayed in contact with many of them, and as far as I can tell they never lost their jobs, or jeopardised their education—as they got older, they simply gave up the drug, and now lead fairly safe and steady lives.

I am reminded of a passage from William Burroughs' *Naked Lunch*, where a middle-use opiate user assumes the narrator's role to tell us that in the futuristic dystopian world:

> How low the other junkies, whereas we—WE have this tent and this lamp, and this tent and this lamp and this tent and nice and warm in here and warm nice and IN HERE … IT'S COLD OUTSIDE where the dross eaters and the needle boys won't last two years … But WE SIT HERE and we never increase the DOSE never-never increase the dose, except TONIGHT is a SPECIAL OCCASION.

I have gotten to know one user, while researching this book, who appears to have her life absolutely together—she is articulate, confident, and introspective—and yet she uses meth nearly every weekend. She gets paid very well in a Sydney corporate marketing job, and told me that she uses frequently, sometimes weekly, but has never missed a day of work, doesn't get depressed, and, all-in-all, her usage doesn't have a negative impact on her life. And I believed her—I often had conversations with her online when she was using, and it often took me a long time to notice she was off her face. She was very friendly and very happy when she was using, and although her thoughts moved more quickly than they normally did, she perhaps wasn't quite as sharp as her usual self. She had a tendency to take things very literally, but generally her mind seemed to operate as usual—perhaps even a bit better.

'So why don't you think it's problematic for you?' I asked her.

'Control,' she replied. 'I always take my dose on a Friday. It keeps me awake for two nights, and then I fall asleep on Sunday afternoon.'

'How do you manage to fall asleep on it?'

'My anti-anxiety medication: I don't come down, I float down.'

Her long sleep from Sunday afternoon to Monday morning mitigated the nights she stayed awake. During those two days, she not only had fun, but also cleaned her house, and came up with many new ideas that she would later implement to enhance both her working and leisure life.

I wasn't around Smithy and Beck when they started using crystallised meth during the summer of 2011–12. But I was there when they first got together in 2007, and I lived with them from 2009 to 2011, when they were using speed each week. What I'd noticed about Smithy was that, during the week, if he didn't have any pot when he was coming down off speed, he would just lie in bed, in a catatonic state, and stare at the walls. If his mood was slightly more elevated than this, he would whinge, complain about everything, and not greet you when you walked in the door. Then 'Smithy Super Saturday' would come again, and he would be in your face, saying, 'I used to think you were just Beck's friend, but now I know you and I are friends—fucking great friends, too. Do you want another line?'

As for their relationship, it was never particularly good. Over time, their arguments became a bi-weekly phenomenon. I had also lived with them for a period of just over a year, about six months into their relationship. I remember getting up in the middle of the night to eat some Nutella; all the lights were off, and Smithy was bedded down in the lounge room (like he always did) while Beck was lying down in bed. They were just winding down from an argument.

Randomly, almost as if he was talking in his sleep, Smithy

yelled out, 'You stupid, dirty fucking slap—'

Without taking a breath, Beck responded, 'You worthless, dole-bludging, lazy, drug-fucked fucking piece of turd—'

'Fucking oxygen thief,' he said after a 30-second pause.

I took the Nutella jar, and tiptoed back to my bedroom.

Over time, I got tired of Smithy's sleaziness when he was off his face, as well as of his passive-aggression when he was coming down. Beck, too, could be extremely trying during the week, screaming at her kids first thing in the morning, and going into crying fits over (apparently) nothing. One day, Smithy and I got into an argument that ended in a physical fight; after that, I didn't see them for another two years. This was the 2011–13 period, when they started using meth. Once they started using, Smithy began committing crimes, his moods became intolerably chaotic, his breath turned rancid and a front tooth fell out, and their arguing got worse. One night, he and Beck had an altercation, during which, according to Beck, she hit him first with her fists and then with a toaster. Smithy had a restraining order issued against her. She got her own place just around the corner, and they started talking again. They were using meth daily by this point—unlike their use of speed, which had been weekly.

Eventually, I started talking to Beck again, and then Smithy. The first night I saw him after our long break (and after he'd started taking crystal meth), he looked noticeably different—he'd gone from looking like a knockabout, 'you beaut', working-class bloke to a grubby criminal. He wore black clothes, had spots on his face, and that prominent missing front tooth. We never mentioned what happened between us the day of the fight—'blokes get over things, blokes don't hold grudges'—and we managed to form a new friendship, stronger than the one we had before.

I tell this story to demonstrate that although Beck and Smithy weren't a clean, nice, problem-free couple, meth *did* ramp up the extent to which their worst sides featured in their lives. Beck became more moody and more verbally abusive to her kids; her tantrums shifted up a gear from yelling to violent outbursts. Smithy's sleaziness became a full-time obsession; his threats to punch me, and others, in the face were almost constant. His paranoia about being ripped off slipped into psychosis at times. Once he started taking meth, he ended up taking so many days off work that his boss told him he should take a permanent vacation. When he went into Centrelink to apply for the dole, they took one look at him and suggested he apply for the Disability Support Pension instead.

Smithy and Beck's descent into problematic meth use had a long, perhaps sequential history, and was often simply dictated by the availability of the drug. All things considered, however, there can be little question that the drug made their lives less stable, and made both of them more prone to violence.

It is important to note that not all meth users become violent. Many meth users already have a history of violence, and many people commit violence when they are not on meth. Others claim to have been on meth when they committed a crime, when, in fact, they weren't. Still, there is little doubt that one of the biggest problems of meth is its apparent relationship with violent behaviour. Indeed, there is a whole body of research that has been conducted in Australia showing that aggression, violent behaviour, and violent crimes are relatively common among chronic illicit methamphetamine users. In 2014, Rebecca McKetin et al. published a study in the journal published by the Society for the Study of Addiction, 'Does methamphetamine use increase violent behaviour? Evidence from a prospective longitudinal study'. The study concluded that, taking into account other variables—such as a person's pre-morbid tendency for violent acts—there was 'a clear dose-response increase in violent behaviour when participants were using methamphetamine compared to when they were not using the drug. This effect was especially large for frequent methamphetamine use (16-plus days of use in the past month), which increased the odds of violent behaviour 10-fold.'

Dr McKetin, who first started studying the link between amphetamines and psychosis when she was doing her PhD in the mid-1990s—long before anybody else in Australia had researched this correlative—told me that:

> We know that people with schizophrenia have too much dopamine in their brain. Meth increases dopamine, and this causes an imbalance—resulting in too little serotonin, our mood regulator, and too much noradrenaline, our 'fight or flight' chemical. Meth has a clear correlation to very violent behaviour. Part of the reason people act violently when they are on the drug is the chemical interaction it causes: low serotonin levels are associated with aggressive behaviour. So, in the end, people are paranoid from too much dopamine, irritable from low serotonin, and overhyped—all at once.

In my experience, the comedown seems to be a particularly high-risk time for violent thoughts to arise. For me, they usually came as a result of psychotic episodes where I felt the need to defend myself from a perceived mob-attack. Research from the United States suggests that between one-quarter and one-third of meth users engage in violent acts while intoxicated or withdrawing from the drug. I wonder how many more contemplate it, or find that violence makes its way into their never-ending vortex of sexual fantasies.

Studies have also shown that meth reduces impulse control and inhibitions, while increasing the likelihood of psychotic episodes; psychotic patients are in turn more likely to be violent than other psychiatric patients. That said, McKetin's 2014 study showed that feelings of violence during the meth rollercoaster have also been found to exist independently of psychotic delusions.

While I have to admit to getting into the odd fight before I became a meth addict, I had never before experienced such moments of blood lust. On ice, I had moments when the ground seemed to split in front of me, when meaning changed, and I experienced what felt like aberrant, ancient, repressed impulses. In those moments, inflicting pain felt like an exciting, transgressive act of destiny, where somehow all the pain, oppression, and condescension I had experienced as a human, and especially as a gay man, could be overcome by a single, spectacular act of cruelty perpetrated on another person. That person's feelings seemed positively inconsequential to the excitement of doing harm.

McKetin's research has also shown that up to 25 per cent of regular users experience psychosis, and that overall about 13 per cent of users report that they've experienced some kind of psychotic episode while on meth. 'One of the most common psychotic fantasies that people tend to have is that they are being watched,' McKetin said. 'For some reason a lot of meth users think there are secret cameras in the house or that the government is spying on them.'

McKetin explained that as many as half of current meth users have previously experienced mental-health problems and taken medication for this condition—most commonly for anxiety, depression, and psychosis.

Yet, at the same time, she told me, 'Our research tends to show that those who experience meth-psychosis rarely have any personal or family history of schizophrenia.'

McKetin told me that the less talked-about, but more common, problem for meth users was mild to moderate depression that often lingered for a long time after someone stopped using, making a relapse more likely. What is not clear is whether a person's depression or suicidal thoughts are caused by the prolonged use of meth, or whether some people who take meth are self-medicating their pre-existing depression. It seems unlikely we will ever have a clear-cut answer to such a complex question, although one 2012 University of Melbourne research project did find that '72 per cent of participants reported that methamphetamine use preceded the onset of mental health problems'.

It would seem that the longer-running risk of meth use is depression and anxiety. Research by Dr Nicole Lee (associate professor at the National Centre for Education and Training on Addiction at Flinders University and adjunct associate professor at the National Drug Research Institute) and her colleagues has found that among 126 Australians who used varying levels of methamphetamine over a certain period of time, 69 per cent had been diagnosed or treated by a doctor for a mental-health problem, most frequently for depression (50 per cent) and anxiety (29 per cent).

Yet, these facts beg an obvious chicken-and-egg question. It seems quite likely that a person who is already down in the dumps (or anxious, or stressed) would take the drug. Meth has quite specific effects—it doesn't bring the connectedness or light-heartedness associated with marijuana, ecstasy, and LSD, but it can make you feel as if you are living in a 1980s TV advertisement, where you have success, friends, boundless energy, endless sunshine, and instant gratification. It makes all your dreams come true, while you become your ego-ideal: an experience I call 'Fantasia'.

In Fantasia, you are not just more successful and powerful than in your wildest dreams, you are the most successful and the most powerful. In my experience, crystal meth provides you with something that is increasingly rare in modern life—it enables you to live in the moment, right-now-in-that-moment when nothing else matters. Meth gives its users many things that seem lacking in our mainstream culture: a chance for unconventional thinking, and a window to mysticism, ritualistic spirituality, drama, and intimacy. These experiential aspects of meth lend themselves to some important cultural analysis: it is the perfect drug in a society where happiness, individual freedom, productivity, and self-esteem are our ultimate goals, but where loneliness, a loss of connection, exhaustion, and insatiable, inexplicable feelings of failure often reign. It is a synthetic drug for a synthetic culture: a modern-day nerve tonic for a 24-hour society. It is an anti-anxiety drug in the age of anxiety: a depression-busting, awe-inspiring chemical that brings a tribe, adventure, and excitement to an often monotonous, uneventful suburban life lacking in community, fun, and meaning. Crystal meth, therefore, has much to offer somebody who is feeling disenchanted with themselves and the modern world—though it can simultaneously inflict the same egomaniacal, lonely, deluded misery that you are trying to escape.

For me—someone who used crystal meth and had a history, and indeed a family history, of both psychosis and addiction—I found that, after a while, life stopped seeming interesting when I was not on meth. In his book *Memoirs of an Addicted Brain: a neuroscientist examines his former life on drugs*, developmental neuroscientist Marc Lewis explains how taking crystal meth gradually seemed to take the kick out of everyday waking life:

> [T]he subterfuge of drugs like methamphetamine culminates in one brilliant trick: the message of meth is that goals don't matter anymore. When engorged on dopamine, the ventral striatum acts as if it's pursuing goals and gloriously, magnificently, achieving them. Yet there are no goals. The excitement is bogus. It's free. It's detached from any actual internal desires or external accomplishments.

I remain deeply sceptical, for several reasons, about casual users who say that meth isn't harming them. First, they may not recognise the harm that is being done (and the idea that a person couldn't be harmed by their drug use because they still work and remain productive really does make me squirm). Second, they may recognise it, but not want to admit it. Third, they may be in a state of denial about how much they are using. Last, one consequence of meth use—even of the kind that cannot be termed addiction—is that people will defend the drug because they want to keep the drug in their lives. Their brains have become so convinced it is good for them that they will use any justification to keep using it, even if it does not appear to be benefiting them, even if it appears to be causing them harm, or, even at the very least, if it is not allowing them to live life to the full or take pleasure in other things.

For me (as for Marc Lewis), the risk of using meth even occasionally is that you stop striving for new goals or new life-experiences that give you the same kind of thrill. Meth attacks your ability to reason, your sense of time, your counting skills—I admire anybody who *is* able to control their use of it. Indeed, the notion that meth use can be non-problematic or even life-enhancing must be tempered by the fact that the drug wears down your self-awareness. Meth is not unlike the bite of the blue-ring octopus, whose poison is worse than its bite: it takes quite some time to realise you have been poisoned. With meth, you can go on functioning and feeling while addiction wraps itself around your body and mind.

Ms Trish Quibell from Berry Street South services in Shepparton told the Victorian parliamentary inquiry:

A lot of our young people would not see themselves as having an addiction; they would completely deny that they have an addiction. That would be prevalent regardless of what strata of society you come from. Most people do not believe they have got an addiction until something hits them and they have hit rock bottom.

With more than a bit of uncertainty floating around my mind about these issues, I decided to ring Dr Nicole Lee to ask some of these questions, knowing that she has a reputation for being fair, centrist, open-minded, and compassionate. In addition to her positions at Flinders University and the National Drug Research Institute, Lee is a practising clinical psychologist. In 2012, she co-edited Australia's most extensive academic book on amphetamines, and her consultancy company, LeeJenn Health Consultants, was hired by the Victorian parliament as part of its inquiry to provide answers to some of the trickiest questions about methamphetamine use in the community.

Lee, a friendly and gentle-sounding person who spent much of our interview listening closely to my questions before giving long, considered answers, told me that she believes there are three broad types of users: acute—who are what we might term meth addicts, and use upwards of once a week; long term—who use intermittently over a long period of time, or go on binges before getting clean in a fairly constant cycle; and occasional users—users who use very, very occasionally, sometimes as infrequently as once a year. To this, she added the caveat that 'unlike many other drugs where addiction is black and white, meth use occurs along a complex and varied continuum'.

So if we are able to draw something of a contingent, cautious line between addicts and non-addicts, where do we go with the question of harm? Does the occasional user risk becoming depressed, anxious, or losing enthusiasm for life?

Lee told me that there is a risk,

but that the risk of occasional users getting any of the serious mental-health issues are very low. It's the long-term users who

we often worry about because they always run the risk of
becoming an acute user … it can also be very difficult for people
to recognise their depression is being caused by their meth use,
and what our research also indicates is that there is often a five-
year gap between when people first develop problematic use and
when they first seek treatment.

And, of course, there is always the risk that when people
report their drug use to a researcher—particularly if they want
reasons to continue their meth use—they will both understate
how much they are using, and overstate the positive impact it is
having on their life.

I also called Neil Mellnor, drug counsellor and lecturer at the
University of Sunshine Coast, who told me he thinks there are
three ways in which people go from being a meth user to being
a meth addict:

1. They drift slowly into ice, and unexpectedly become
   addicted.
2. They take ice without understanding its full effects, prefer
   using meth to other drugs because its effects last longer,
   and eventually become addicted.
3. They are in a scene where it is acceptable or 'cool', and
   begin using it as a drug of choice.

'When somebody gets too far into meth addiction, daily life
just starts to feel like a grind,' he said. 'They prefer being on meth
than not. Their health starts to decline, their everyday reality feels
less and less tolerable—they start to struggle financially. Then a
classic addiction-cycle starts—the worse life gets, the more drugs
they take, and the more drugs they take, the worse their life gets.'

Even in retrospect, I have trouble piecing together exactly
when the bit-of-fun use ended for me, and the serious, abusive

use began. I can see only the after-effect, not the exact moment when I slipped from user to addict. In his book *Crazy Town: money, marriage, meth*, former addict Sterling R. Braswell compares the experience of being an addict to being Gollum from *Lord of the Rings*: 'We forgot the taste of bread, the sound of trees, the softness of the wind, we even forgot our own name.' My time in the house became a mess of sped-up time and drawn-out days, of coming down in bed, of blackouts, and of excursions into make-believe. The defining moment may have taken place when I started shoplifting food; the day I thought everyone was going to kill me; the day of my bloody needle-stick injury; the day I started using two days in a row; the moments I spent fantasising about my next high while walking through the homogenised streets of inner Sydney. It may have come around the time I began having a recurring dream of walking along a field, and suddenly realising I was surrounded by steep drops, and was desperately hanging on, so as not to fall. When I had these dreams at Smithy's, I eventually decided to let go, and enjoy the exhilaration and thrill of the fall. Falling can be joyful, even if you know that death awaits, and especially when you are so tired of holding on, and so sick of being scared.

Even still, I have met users who suggest that meth makes them better people, and improves their lives; people who think the drug brings them experience and thrills that are beyond the normal, limited realm of human experience. They think meth makes them perform better, think better, and become better, faster, more evolved human beings.

'I cannot imagine living without it,' one user told me. 'I get so much done, I work so much out when I am on it. Actually, I don't think I am that different when I use it, and often people around me can't even tell.'

Many people simply think that meth isn't affecting them at all. Apart from the possibility they are delusional, perhaps this also reflects the way new technologies have come to play an apparently inconspicuous role in our lives, while at the same time radically altering the experience and understanding of our own nature. Meth is a wholly synthetic drug, one of over twenty-million chemicals that have been created in the past hundred years, and it is often, and ironically, providing a pathway for many of us to discover the beast of yesteryear.

## Chapter Three

# Converging paths

THE ORIGINS OF meth can be traced to the chemical-research labs of nineteenth-century Japan. The late nineteenth century was a time of considerable scientific advance: medicine was riding high on the discoveries of microbes, vaccines, anaesthetics, painkillers, and the realisation that humans had powerful biochemical signals called 'hormones'. Scientists around the world had set about trying to find a synthetic compound of the human hormone adrenaline, which was at that time particularly expensive to make because it had to be extracted from cow glands. Attention turned to the Ephedra plant, an unremarkable-looking organism that grows in sandy soils in sun-drenched environments, and that had been used for centuries in Chinese medicine. Its purported energy- and mood-enhancing effects came to be seen as a potential base for a new adrenaline-like product, as scientists believed it held the secrets to human fatigue and the common cold.

Dr Nagai Nagayoshi commenced work on his study of ephedra after returning from Berlin University in 1883. Nagayoshi was wide-eyed and impeccably dressed, and his lab at the Tokyo Imperial University consisted of wooden tables, with chemicals held in bottles like old-fashioned lolly jars. Like all lab researchers at the time, he did not wear lab coats or masks to work, but dressed as if he were working in an office.

Nagayoshi spent two years studying the plant, eventually finding the active alkaloid, ephedrine. Amphetamine sulphate (not meth, but similar) was actually the first compound to be developed, a few years earlier. It was made accidentally by the Romanian chemist Lazăr Edeleanu when he was trying to synthesise the world's first amphetamine (speed, not meth) while making new fabric dyes. Eventually, Dr Nagayoshi used Edeleanu's formula to synthesise amphetamine from ephedrine, creating a more powerful formula: methamphetamine (powdered meth).

Today, ephedrine and pseudoephedrine are the two most common precursor chemicals used in making crystal meth.

Professor Nicolas Rasmussen from the University of New South Wales writes in his book *On Speed: the many lives of amphetamine* that methamphetamines and amphetamines developed in the tradition of 'old human fantasies of magical cures and elixirs of youth'. He writes that in 'the age of science-based pharmaceuticals … we expect new triumphs of science that, in our lifetime, will eliminate mankind's most ancient enemies — the illnesses that bring pain, sorrow, frailty, and ultimately death'.

Intrigued by this observation, I decided to ring Professor Rasmussen — who has earned, by the way, no less than a PhD from Stanford and a Masters from Cambridge — to find out a bit more about his studious work on the history of the drug. I found him to be a fast-talking, fastidiously helpful American who stops every now and then to ask — as a matter of genuine courtesy — 'Are you following?'

Rasmussen's history lesson taught me a few things — first, unlike cocaine or heroin, meth is a purely synthetic substance. Second, methamphetamine differs from amphetamine only in the addition of a methyl group on the chemical chain; the difference of just one extra carbon — 'meth' (actually methyl) — is what makes taking meth feel as if you're taking off in aeroplane, and makes taking speed feel as if you're 'merely' travelling in a V8. Third, that perhaps it is no accident that methamphetamine was born in the age of scientific advances, the rise of the corporation, and the rise of a liberal society in which there is a perpetual promise that hard work will pay off.

In April 1981, Rob Smith was seven years old. Waking up one morning in his cosy three-bedroom brick house, on the foothills of Melbourne's tree fern-covered Dandenong Ranges, his ears fixed on a strange howl coming from somewhere inside the house.

He followed the sound. His feet tapped along the cold floorboards, past a picture of a little English cottage surrounded by autumn trees. The path took him to his mother's room. The door was half-open, and his mother was sobbing on the end of her bed, her head resting on her left hand. Feeling his stare, she sat up, wiping her face with her hands. She smiled at her son, saying in her soft voice: 'Hello, darling, how ya feelin' this morning? You're awake very early, mate.'

He trotted up to her and wrapped his hands gently around her neck. His face pressed against hers, and he felt the hotness of her tears as they soaked into his skin. She smelt like make-up, hairspray, and sweat. She smelt like his mummy. He didn't understand why she was crying, though, and instinctively he began to sob as well.

'Dad's gone,' she said with a look of anguished, apologetic horror.

She told him to go back to bed. As he lay down, he could hear his mother's howls starting up again, more intensely, and she continued right through the morning.

—

In 1996, two awkward teenagers were sitting by the fire, wrapped in blankets, drinking sugary tea and enjoying each other's company at 2.00am on a Sunday. Those teenagers were Beck and me, and the lounge room was in her parent's musty, homely place in our rough bush-town. Beck had turned off *Rage* over an hour before; the open fire was only just still burning, and fatigue was slowing her monologue and slurring her words.

'Some people are good at sport or maths, some people are pretty,' she explained. 'I don't think I'm good at anything. I was hopeless at netball, I dropped out of school, and the best I ever got was a B. I'm not particularly good-looking, I don't even really have an identity—I'm not really *anyone*. Do you get what I mean?'

Beck continued at length, detailing all the things she wasn't good at before concluding:

'The only thing I am good at is giving people money, and the only time I am happy is when I am sick. I really like *Trainspotting* and *Pulp Fiction*. It's just so cool, and they have so much fun, and I know this sounds really awful, so don't, like, tell anyone this, but I am thinking about becoming like a junkie—it makes you somebody.'

I didn't answer. The fire fizzled out. We both fell asleep.

In 1919, methamphetamine hydrochloride was synthesised by Nagayoshi's protégé, the Japanese pharmacologist Akira Ogata. Ogata was experimenting with Nagayoshi's formula and its base materials when he made a reduction of ephedrine using red phosphorus and iodine, producing the world's first batch of crystallised meth.

Today, the street slang for meth confuses the fact there are actually three distinct formulas: 'speed' (which is amphetamine sulphate); Nagayoshi's 'meth' (which is the powdered meth that has been in Australia since about the mid-1990s); and Ogata's 'ice' (crystallised meth, the drug that is causing all the trouble of late). All three formulas were developed in the late nineteenth or early twentieth century, but they didn't come into pharmaceutical use until the 1920s. When they did so, it was in the context of the creation of pharmaceutical patents, which allowed companies to 'own' some of these formulas and variations of them, and therefore to sell them under specific brand names.

When little Smithy woke the day after he found his mum crying, his dad still wasn't there; nor was he there the next day, nor the one after that. The truth was obvious—his father was gone. For nearly nine months after, while the oval behind his house filled with large puddles and a choir of frogs, which then disappeared again, Rob Smith barely spoke a word. He spent nearly every spare minute lying on his bed, staring at the floor.

His mum increased her work hours as an office manager in a local factory to pay the mortgage. This meant she wasn't there in the morning and she was not usually home when he got back from school. But on the weekends, when she saw him lying on the bed, she would ask him what was wrong. 'Nothing,' he would say. 'Just tired.' When she gazed at him, she saw a littler version of her husband: the same brown hair, blue eyes, and oval face; the football watching, the cricket playing, and the fart jokes.

The months he spent in silence in his room were countered by her with toys, lollies, and chocolate. She enrolled him in football and cricket. And bit by bit, little Smithy came back to life, with a deeper, darker sense of humour, and a new taste for naughty things. He started watching football and cricket again, and got used to watching them by himself. He started socialising again like mad, with a particular taste for pranks and ridiculous jokes. He was never lacking in friends at school. He was 'one of the boys', and all his mates played on the same football team as him. He admired alpha males, and had a soft spot for the underdog. Smithy remembers going to a friend's house, and overhearing the boy's mother talking about him before he walked in the door.

'He's a no-hoper,' she said. 'That's what happens when you don't have a father to set you right.'

He decided not to go in, and felt upset for a good week after. The words played on his mind for months, until he decided, 'Well, I guess if I'm no good, I may as well have fun.' Perhaps, he decided, not having any expectations meant one thing—freedom.

As he a teenager, he loved parties. He liked to get drunk—he liked spin-the-bottle and truth-or-dare. At fourteen, he dropped out of school. He would spend many of his days getting drunk or stoned. Later, he'd be introduced to speed by a 37-year-old neighbour he was having an affair with. He loved the energy, the confidence, the sense of fullness and cohesion he got from speed—the feeling of a never-ending party.

For thirty years after they were made, nobody knew what to do with meth, crystal meth, and speed. Then along came Gordon Alles, a 6-foot-something alpha American male who had completed a PhD at the California Institute of Technology, where he had attempted to find a synthetic version of human insulin. He went to work for a big pharma company, and spent most of his downtime working on a new cold-and-flu formulation. In 1928, he independently resynthesised the original amphetamine formula (that is, amphetamine sulphate) and discovered its wide-ranging effects on the human nervous system (this was speed, not meth, and Alles didn't create it—he just found out how it works). In early self-experiments, he would report a feeling of 'self-exhilaration'; its results on asthma were mixed, but its effect on moods was exemplary. Nonetheless, he found it could also be used as a bronchial dilator, and sold his patent on the formulation to the big American pharmaceutical company Smith, Kline, & French (SKF). SKF then went on to sell the amphetamine under the brand name 'Benzedrine' in pills and inhalers. It was first sold as a decongestant, but by the 1930s, the company was promoting it as a treatment for 33 different ailments, from alcoholism to erectile dysfunction. SKF also marketed it to expectant mothers for weight-loss, extra energy, and as an anti-depressant.

While meth was more powerful than speed, pharmaceutical companies and scientists were unable to find a way to tweak its formula enough to fit the legal criteria to make it an 'original discovery' and therefore eligible to receive a proprietary patent. Benzedrine also received support from the American Psychological Association, which advised psychiatrists to start prescribing the drug to certain patients. This marked the start of a 20-year period in which amphetamines became the most commonly prescribed anti-depressant in the western world.

In post-depression America, speed (Benzedrine) became the obvious choice for a world in which things were moving faster, and individual unhappiness was seen as a purely personal medical problem in what was a booming economy. In fact, the 1930s were the start of amphetamine's golden age. Not only were the side effects of amphetamines unknown, but they were developed at a time when the pharmaceutical industry was largely unregulated, and amphetamines could be purchased without a prescription over the counter at a variety of different stores. People even started getting high while they were, well, already high: Benzo inhalers started appearing on Pan Am flight menus in the 1940s, alongside cigarettes, drinks, and cocktails.

Australia was also quick to embrace these new products. On 4 August 1936, Mt Gambier's *The Border Mail* published an article titled 'New Drug will Banish Shyness' that referenced a 'new drug called Benzedrine, which raises the blood pressure and is also thought to cure depression and shyness'. The *Adelaide*

*Advertiser* followed on 28 August 1936, in an article titled 'New Drug for Happiness', in which the journalist reported that 'Dr Gordon Alles has found a new drug, according to the latest messages from England, which may result in happiness pills becoming a reality, and be able to turn melancholia into cheerfulness within an hour. Moreover, it is claimed that this new drug, Benzedrine, is supposed not to be habit-forming, and not to have dangerous after-effects.'

Evidently, there was unmitigated optimism about speed when it first hit the market legally. There were over 70 articles published about the drug in Australia throughout the late 1930s and early 1940s, all of which talked up the newfound happiness pill that also made you smarter. No endorsement, though, compared to the one published in Adelaide's *The Mail* on 15 May 1937: 'Soon We Will All Be Brilliant' ran the headline to the short article, reporting that while the drug might be addictive, it also led to more fluent and convincing speech.

For a long time, you could buy meth in Australian pharmacies. For a while, you didn't even need a prescription to buy it. Meth was often sold under the brand name 'Methedrine', which was sometimes advertised in magazines and newspapers. One Methedrine ad from 1948 shows an illustration of a smiling woman, with the tagline 'Methedrine is good for creating the Right Attitude'. Other ads suggested that the drug could 'increase your optimism', help you lose weight ('help *her* resist temptation'), and relieve fatigue. Syndrox, another legal powdered-meth formulation, was — according to the ad — for the overweight 'patient who is all flesh and no will power'. Long before Prozac and anti-psychotics, meth — under its various brand names — was prescribed by psychiatrists as an anti-depressant, and you could even get an intravenous Methedrine injection from the doctor if you felt you needed it.

During the Second World War, meth and benzos were used

widely by soldiers across all sides to boost military performance. This led to an excess of production, and to many soldiers returning to the US, Germany, Japan, and the UK with leftover meth and speed — thereby leading to one of the world's first black markets in amphetamines.

In his book *No Speed Limit: the highs and lows of meth*, Frank Owen says that the 1940s and 1950s were a time when 'there was a naïve belief that science and technology could solve all our problems ... Television and magazines bombarded consumers with images for a perfect lifestyle, especially for women, a number of whom felt trapped and alienated by this often-lonely new reality. Amphetamine appeared tailor-made for this new way of living — a synthetic drug for a synthetic environment.' In *Speed*, Professor Rasmussen tells how 'President John F. Kennedy received regular injections of a methamphetamine, together with vitamins and hormones, from a German-trained physician named Max Jacobson. Jacobson would go on to treat Cecil B. DeMille, Alan Jay Lerner, Truman Capote, Tennessee Williams, and the Rolling Stones.'

However, by the late 1940s Benzedrine was becoming associated with crime, counter-culture, and deviancy. In 1948, a New South Wales man was jailed for vagrancy (that is to say, poverty), having told the court that he had been taking 200 Benzedrine tablets a day. A few months later, a 47-year-old telegraphist from Burwood, Arthur Haybe, was charged with murder, and told detectives he had used Benzedrine tablets 'to keep himself awake in the early hours of morning' because he believed his wife 'visited a neighbour at night'. Even poor Dr George Basil Goswell, from Walgett, in New South Wales, fell into the trap. He started writing bad cheques after he became addicted to his clinic's Benzedrine tablets. He told the court that he became addicted because of the pressure of work.

By this time, both members of the public and prominent medical authorities were demanding that Benzedrine tablets be made available on prescription only. In October 1948, an unnamed 60-year-old mother of two Benzedrine addicts (aged twenty-six and twenty-eight) publicly urged effective control of Benzedrine sales. She told reporters that her sons were taking up to 80 tablets a day, and said, 'Benzedrine is slowly murdering my boys before my eyes. It is heart-breaking.' Her calls were welcomed and supported by both New South Wales police and the New South Wales public health director-general. Within a few years, and across all states, Benzedrine could only be obtained with a legal prescription. However, its less understood and more powerful older brother — Methedrine — was still widely available.

By the mid-1960s, edgy Australian partygoers were taking Methedrine in the bright, new discotheque scene. On 28 June 1967, *The Canberra Times* published an article titled 'Night Spot, a den for drug addicts and criminals', which went on to explain that the Licensing Court had denied a liquor licence to the Catcher Discotheque in Flinders Lane, Melbourne, following reports — among many others — that girls had admitted taking Methedrine and Dexedrine to 'keep dancing or just to stay awake'. Just a few months earlier, 19-year-old Peter Graham Johnson had been described by a magistrate as a 'crazy mixed-up kid' while being sentenced to two years' probation for selling Methedrine at the Catcher.

These were the kinds of events that led to meth becoming more or less illegal by the mid-1970s. By this stage, politicians in both Australia and the United States were making more and more noise about the damage amphetamines were doing to society. After a number of drugged drivers were left unprosecuted, New South Wales health minister Harry Jago moved in 1965 to outlaw driving under the influence of Methedrine. Indeed, history should look kindly upon the Liberal member for Fuller who, four years later—and several years before a global, UN-led push to do the same—moved to restrict the illegal sale of amphetamines. Jago would eventually usher in new legislation requiring any person making or distributing amphetamines to maintain a register recording all drugs supplied or manufactured. While Jago was well-meaning and forward thinking, the problem of fraud remained an obvious blind spot for this legislation. As has been a constant theme in history, greater regulation did little to sway the growth of the amphetamine black market. In 1969 alone, there were 230 robberies of chemists and warehouses throughout Australia to obtain narcotics and amphetamines. In a letter published in *The Medical Journal of Australia* in September 1967, prominent psychiatrist Cedric Swanton wrote that 'the extent of the consumption of amphetamines by the community might be gleaned from the fact that quite recently one of the drug companies' premises was broken into and robbed of 130,000 "methedrine" tablets.'

Swanton's views were quickly becoming mainstream among global elites, and things were set to change. The US government stepped in to put a stop to it all by enacting the Controlled Substances Act in 1970, which all but entirely restricted the sale of meth. The United Nations followed with a major international treaty: the 1971 Convention on Psychotropic Substances. Australia would soon follow America and the UN's lead by enacting the 1976 Psychotropic Substances Act, banning the sale of most meth and amphetamine products.

Meth production moved to the black market, and in particular biker gangs, which would later join up with Mexican cartels.

If I had my time again, on that night of self-loathing and pregnant pauses, when Beck announced her perverse ambition to become a drug addict, I would have told her that she had many, many talents. That she could easily be a scientist or a comedy writer. She, like her dad, was a natural caregiver; she could have been a magnificent social worker or community builder. It was only that she lacked the resilience, self-belief, and patience to work at her talents long enough for them to develop into skills. What needed to be said was that people become good at things through willpower and persistence, that she was a victim of her own self-fulfilling prophecy, and that she was young and had a lifetime to make good.

Ironically, at that stage I harboured ambitions of being a psychologist who lived in the mountains, wore tweed coats, had a big bookshelf, and lived by myself. It didn't occur to me that I lacked the ability to say the right thing at the right moment. Drugs vaguely interested me, but I was determined to become a stuffy intellectual—I never imagined I would have the social skills, or the nihilism, to last in drug culture. I had gotten rotten drunk at parties as an early teenager, and always regretted it—on a number of levels—the next day. I liked sitting at home alone, doing my own thing; at other times, I spent time with Mum and her friends.

I remember growing up feeling that I was someone special, and Mum was always telling me she thought I'd grow up to be somebody important. I remember the private drama, tennis, and singing lessons: the wild aspirations, and the triumphs and failures that followed. I remember Mum reading a book with me out loud, over and over again. The book was called *The Little Engine That Could*.

I grew up in a semi-rural area with a golf course and patches of wet, rocky, fern-covered bush. My mind might be playing tricks on me, but I remember my childhood as a series of happy, shining moments connected by long walks through the bush with my Labrador, Daisy. She would always lead the way: we would find rabbits, foxes, echidnas, and wombats. (Apparently she thought these creatures were playmates rather than food, and whenever we found an echidna she would take one sniff and go running away.) I lived in a neighbourhood with half a dozen boys my age, who would often accompany us. We would build cubbies, get chased by bulls, and swing off a rope tied to a tree into a lake—which was once the town's source of water—that had its own waterfall, surrounded by tall tree-ferns and a little apple orchid. I remember summer evenings at dusk, playing tennis with Dad, netball matches with my sister in the backyard, endless one-on-one basketball tournaments with my next-door neighbour, extravagant Christmas mornings, and 'going to war' with the other boys. During these games, allegiances were always changing, and they usually climaxed in an exhilarating punch-up. Of course, we all became friends again the following week, and then we'd turn again, or pick a new opponent when we got bored.

I was naughty in school; I got into trouble a lot. I wasn't allowed to backchat at home, so I did so at school. I always had trouble concentrating, I often felt bored, I made stupid mistakes, and I was usually desperate to fit in, and put on a show. I have never taken criticism or rejection well. I always wanted everybody to like me.

Meanwhile, Beck was making her way through the final acts of her teenage years, changing her costume from hippie to cowgirl to gangster chick along the way. Beck lived in Cockatoo, a bush town about ten minutes from my straight-laced hometown of Emerald, and about an hour-and-a-half's drive from Melbourne. Cockatoo, and many of its residents, had been burnt to a crisp during the Ash Wednesday fires. A series of extremely cheap houses, some actual housing commission homes, hippies, and criminals arose from the ashes—a group affectionately (and sometimes not-so-affectionately) known as the 'Cockatoo Scum'. In Cockatoo, there were always bizarre crimes being committed and weird drugs being indulged in, strange ideas floating around, and people who looked like they had been born as the result of incest, or as if their mothers had taken thalidomide. Cockatoo was the place my mum told me to stay away from; Cockatoo was my kind of place.

Before I ever spoke to Beck, I knew her by reputation. She was commonly known as an easy root, an underachiever, and a sook; a bit clingy, but also a genuinely nice person who wouldn't hurt a fly. She was certainly a drifter, a magnet for virtual stray cats (and, later in life, actual stray cats), and her dress sense left some ambiguity as to whether she was a nonconformist by accident or design. At first, she was as fascinating as a car wreck. But as we became closer, she seemed to be the only person at our school who seemed interested in anything other than cars, football, and social hierarchies. Beck told me that people liked to scapegoat, exclude, and tease her for their own entertainment. She told me she was teased for being poor in primary school (or, more particularly, because her mother made her clothes), and in Year 7 her parents received a series of anonymous phone calls from giggling, boyish voices asking if they could speak with the 'BI-LO bitch'. Occasionally this would bring her to tears, but more often she invented cutting private jokes about the perpetrators, and did excellent, abstract impersonations of them when in peak form.

I was sure she was going to prove them all wrong one day; she was one of the deepest people I had ever met.

The 1971 UN convention became a watershed moment in our global problem with meth abuse. During the 1980s, the US government restricted access to and increased penalties for possession of P2P—the key ingredient for making meth. But such is the plight of good intentions that this only resulted in bikie gangs discovering they could make meth from ephedrine, resulting in a more powerful formula that could be easily obtained from Mexican labs that professed to be making the substance purely for legal cold-and-flu tablets. As amphetamines came back into fashion, with ecstasy and MDMA pills spreading around nightclubs and raves around the world in the late 1980s, crystal meth gradually got a stranglehold on a small proportion of America's population. In a survey conducted in 2012, approximately 1.2 million Americans reported having used methamphetamine in the previous year, while 440,000 reported using the drug in the previous month. This was a smaller user percentage of the population than when the drug had been legally prescribed — but the legal Methedrine, Desoxyn, and Syndrox had been made from the powdered formula, whereas crystal meth was the substance dominating the American black market.

The rise of crystal meth in Australia would follow the same pattern, albeit a few decades later. Why so much later? Well, Australia's biggest drug problem from the 1960s right until the new millennium was heroin, due to the island nation's proximity to poppy fields across South-East Asia.

Like most people in the mid-1990s in Australia, Beck and I had never heard of or seen meth. In fact, the data shows that from the 1970s through to the 1980s, amphetamine use sat at around 4 per cent of the population — most of those were using amphetamine sulphate, and most had had it prescribed to them. It was a cheap, working-class drug, different in both its cultural identity and chemistry from cocaine. MDMA (ecstasy) would also make its way to Australian shores in the 1970s. MDMA, which is both an amphetamine and a psychedelic drug, appears to have been brought here from India by a religious group called 'The Orange People', who used the drug as part of their mystic process, whereby they saw sex as a path to enlightenment. Some psychiatrists in Australia, as part of their treatment for post-traumatic stress disorder, even used ecstasy on their patients, before the practice was made illegal by the Australian government in 1985. Speed, and in some cases meth, was made in clandestine labs here and there across the nation, but hardly any Australians used either drug throughout the 1980s. The first batches of powdered methamphetamine arrived on our shores in the early 1990s; a minor rise in use followed, but none of this, as far as we know, was crystal meth. Government research from that time showed past-year use of amphetamines was less than 1 per cent in 1993 and 1995; lifetime use was around 4–5 per cent. The use of amphetamines was largely restricted, it seemed, to nightclubbers, and people wanting to increase their work hours and output. In the 1980s, in 'relaxed Australia', heroin remained king; some estimates suggest that there were as many 172,000 people injecting heroin in Australia in 1986 alone.

So, while the drug barely registered a ripple here, it was a different tale overseas. By the late 1980s, the recipes used by US biker gangs, and the many home-labs that followed, had made their way to parts of South-East Asia. Throughout the early 1990s, crystal meth was manufactured en masse in China, becoming the most widely abused drug in Burma and Japan, and the second most widely abused drug in the Philippines. When the US government then moved to restrict ephedrine, the bikers started using pseudoephedrine to make their meth, resulting in a more powerful formula again. More importantly, the formula was easy to make, and home labs began popping up all over the US.

A few years earlier, an unknown chemist in Hawaii had manufactured a smokeable form of crystal meth. This led to full-scale production on the US island, with the nearby nations of Taiwan and Korea soon learning the recipe and following suit. These trends alarmed many crime authorities here in Australia. In 1989, South Sydney drug detective Brent Martin told journalists he thought the Asian experience showed that meth might replace cocaine as Australia's choice stimulant. Come 1991, and Customs and the Australian Federal Police (AFP) followed suit, warning of the new threat of a drug called 'ice', and lobbying the federal government to develop a campaign to stop its spread. Even so, the drug either continued to fly completely under the radar, or perhaps it didn't even make it to our shores for at least another four years—nobody quite knows. What we do know is that the increase in the supply and use of methamphetamine in Australia appears to have begun around the mid- to late 1990s, while the more potent forms of 'base' and 'ice' methamphetamine were first detected in 1999.

Also in 1991, the same year that the US government gave speed to its war pilots in the first Gulf War, two momentous events occurred sequentially in Smithy's life. He was eighteen, driving home one night on a near-empty Burwood Highway under orange lights through never-ending suburbia. He had just sold some pot and a bit of speed at a friend's house, and Led Zeppelin was blaring through his speakers as he bopped along to the rhythm of the road, sipping on a VB, the stale smell of cigarette smoke drifting around him. When he caught a reflection of himself in the rear-view mirror, he realised he was smiling like a Cheshire cat. But the next time he looked in the mirror, he saw blue lights flashing. Smithy was arrested, and charged with drug trafficking. The second event occurred after his mum contacted his father about the charges. After twelve years of complete silence, his father responded, paid for a lawyer, and told Smithy that everything would sort itself out. And it did: Smithy was put on a good-behaviour bond without a conviction.

A new pattern had been set: Smithy—quite a likeable person for the most part, I might add—would work at odd labouring jobs, where he'd do pot and speed all day, until he found the speed more interesting. He would then leave his job to become a small-time drug dealer. He never made a profit, but the trade meant he had a steady supply of drugs, and of people—including women—knocking on the door. When he ran out of drugs, his phone often fell silent, leading him to lie on the floor when he was coming down, staring at the wall and thinking, *They are not my real friends, they are not my real friends, they are not my real friends—nobody visits me when I've run out of drugs.* He would feel miserable, alone and unloved, until the next speed delivery, after which his house would once again be full of people and grog, and the rooms would be filled with the warm sound of his deep, wheezy cackle.

The mid-1990s were also a time when different kinds of social misfits were working out how to make something of themselves, outside the boundaries and expectations of acceptable society. As *Breaking Bad* would later teach us—in spectacularly entertaining fashion—meth production and distribution could bring the kind of wealth that people working in everyday jobs could only dream of.

Before this time, the passing-on of meth recipes was limited to physical delivery and word of mouth. This all changed, of course, with the advent of the internet. Soon there were dozens of websites publishing the biker method for making methamphetamine hydrochloride (crystal meth) using pseudoephedrine. Other recipes also made their way to Australian living rooms. The results of meth production would show up in some very random places. In 1995, in the stunning inland Sunshine Coast town of Gympie, a place full of palm trees and beautiful old buildings—surrounded by tree-covered hills—layman Dale Francis Drake made meth using an incredibly simple formula. He, in turn, showed various other people how to make meth by this method. Soon, meth cooks weren't rare commodities, but simple, everyday crooks who just needed to be trained. Over the next four years, clandestine labs in the Sunshine Coast would triple, and amphetamine-related hospital admissions in Queensland would skyrocket.

Starting around 1997, Australian bikie gangs, in particular, began making methamphetamine, thereby giving 'speed' — that inferior Romanian sulphate version — the flick. One young man who started to see a cloudy, exciting combination of powdered meth and dollar signs was a 25-year-old truck driver by the name of Richard James Walsh. Walsh left his job in the country town of Maryland, north of Sydney, to take up a very different sort of heavy lifting — he became a meth dealer to bikies. A heavily built, fearsome-looking bloke with dark skin, a goatee, and five earrings in his left ear, he was already a member of the Nomads bikie gang. With meth becoming increasingly popular around Sydney, Walsh would travel to a manufacturer in Queensland about every three weeks to purchase several pounds of the drug. His business grew quickly. As a dealer at the top of the chain, Walsh also quickly ascended the leadership ladder to become a senior figure within the Nomads. Over time, he formed an important relationship with one particular cook on the Gold Coast — Todd Little, president of the Nomad's Gold Coast chapter. Little, despite being nearly illiterate, had taught himself how to cook meth. Little got his precursor material by paying people to go from chemist to chemist purchasing huge quantities of Sudafed, from which he would then extract pseudoephedrine.

Over the space of four years, Little would make no less than 19 kilograms of powdered meth for Walsh, who in turn passed the gear on to dealers who distributed it further down the chain. Walsh would eventually look beyond Little, and between 1997 and 2001 is estimated to have supplied about 450 kilograms of methamphetamine to the drug markets of Melbourne and Sydney. He would, in the end, play an important role in Australia's first major meth trend — the bikies' involvement in spreading methamphetamine around the nation. By the 2000s, police estimated that Australia's bikie gangs had a 75 per cent control of the meth market.

Like many truck drivers, 37-year-old Darri Haynes took speed to help him get through his shifts. While he didn't understand it at the time, by about 1997 what he was taking, in fact, was meth. Haynes had been using it to try to get through some extremely tough shifts (which later resulted in his employer being successfully prosecuted in court for having failed to provide safe working conditions). After having driven more than 5,400 kilometres in the last week of August 1999, he called fellow truckie Duncan Mackeller, and told him he was so tired that he was 'even starting to hear voices'.

'I am even talking to them now,' he said.

To which Mackeller replied jokingly, 'As long they don't talk back.'

On 1 September, Haynes's vehicle collided with a truck on the Pacific Highway, near Grafton, in the northern rivers region of New South Wales. The truck veered off the road and caught fire. Haynes took just over three minutes to die after the impact, and was little more than a 'sack of ashes' when emergency crews arrived on the scene.

Things were changing in fits and starts, on the global, local, and individual scales. As Malcolm Knox writes in his book *Scattered: the inside story of ice in Australia*:

Up to 1999, there was still scepticism about the term 'ice'. Many in law enforcement, health and academic research believed that ice was a new dealer's brand name for speed … but it wasn't so. Ice was, in fact, new. A profound revolution was taking place—a revolution in composition, the manufacture, the economics of supply and usage—a true cultural revolution.

By now, Beck had left school and taken a job as a checkout chick in a supermarket. She went on a few minor, joyful fucking sprees, and eventually fell pregnant. At seventeen, in the middle of autumn, she rang me from a drab, deserted children's playground in her hometown, saying she had finally made a decision about whether to keep her baby.

'A baby will be unconditional love,' she said, sounding as if she was blowing out the smoke from a cigarette. 'It's something I've never had from my parents, and something I've never had from all those guys who dumped me. A child loves their parent no matter what, and I really want that. I'm going to have this baby.'

## Chapter Four

# The hazardous bush

ON A BRIGHT spring morning in November 1969, just after 7.00am, 48-year-old Mildred Williams woke up in her musty East Bentleigh home. Her husband, Ronald—who was not usually awake at this hour—was not asleep next to her. She called out for him. Five minutes went past, and she called out again. Mildred pulled herself out of bed, still in her nightdress, and walked around the house. She must have looked in every room twice before finally deciding to venture outside. She called out when she first walked out the back door, and then again when she reached the clothesline halfway up the yard. She headed over to the garage, which was closed up, opened the side door, and found Ron with his back to her, perfectly still, hanging from a steel rafter, his feet a metre off the ground.

In 1942, my grandfather—Ronald Arthur Williams, already married and the father of two children—decided he would enrol in the army. He was signed to the 58/59th Battalion, which fought against the Japanese in New Guinea. He had never been to battle before, and had never left the country. He arrived in New Guinea in October of that year. Two years later, he had some kind of mental breakdown amid the gunfire and the mud and the rain. He was medically discharged with a diagnosis of 'war neurosis' in 1944.

He returned home to Melbourne, where he had six more children—my father was a twin and the second youngest—and they all lived in that cramped, grotty, dark timber-board home in East Bentleigh. Nanna Mildred was an illegal bookie; Pop made sawdust, and sold it to butchers. Dad remembers his father waking up in the middle of the night, screaming over and over that the Japanese were coming. At other times, Pop had waking nightmares where he believed he was still in the war; he would hide in closets and under the bed, as if under attack. When these waking nightmares lasted more than a week, he was put in a mental institution. He seemed to get worse as he got older.

Nobody in my family knows exactly what Pop did in that war. All the older siblings have since died—one from suicide—and so nobody is alive to tell me what he was like before he went to war. A little while ago, I started looking around for a book to read to find out more about the New Guinea war. Many have similar-sounding titles: *Hell's Battlefield* by Phillip Bradley, *The Hard Slog* by Karl James, *Bastard of a Place* by Peter Brune. Eventually, I settled on *The Toughest Fighting in the World,* a book by Australian journalist George Johnson, who was embedded with Australian troops in New Guinea throughout the war. From this book, I would learn that Pop moved from the oak-lined suburbs and often chilly winds of inner Melbourne to the terrible mountains, constant rain, mud, malaria, water snakes, crocodile-infested waters, kamikaze attacks, and sniper's nests of the war. Men would return from mission back to main camp unshaven, with sunken cheeks. When Australians were killed, it was usually right in front of their war mates, sometimes in their arms, and sometimes gradually, after incurring mortal, slow-burn wounds in rugged, remote areas where help could not reach them. Johnson recalls the 'whining drone of Japanese aircraft ... the whistle of bombs descending through the humid blackness of the night, the sullen thunder of high explosive falling around the waterfront'. This was a place where a walk through the jungle—while water-logged, covered in mud, and carrying a heavy backpack—would frequently attract gunfire from an unknown source; each step could be your or your mate's last.

As a child, I knew nothing of this war. I spent hours and hours in a battle-fantasy world in the backyard with toy guns and swords. In my childlike fantasies of war, battles didn't come to an end because you were throwing up, or you'd sprained your ankle, or because you'd started hallucinating, or you couldn't stop crying. When things got awful in *my* war, it was all the more exciting. I always did something heroic to save the day. The battle scenes—as they no doubt were for many other kids playing out these epic fantasies—were movie-like, all encompassing and awesome. To my mind, war was a barrel of monkeys, which both gave me a sense of power and reinforced my idea that the world—even in chaos—flowed with moral righteousness.

Dad was sixteen when his father died. He has nothing positive to say about his upbringing. He recalls the filth of the place most of all: once, when they were cooking a roast, he discovered that a rat was cooking alongside the leg of mutton on the oven's floor. He remembers that all the children slept in the same bed, that he had no shoes or socks, that his feet were cold in the winter. He remembers not being able to read or write at school, and how the teachers called him stupid. When Pop died, Dad still hadn't been taught how to read or write. He had already left school, and was working in a piggery. He worked with a knife mainly. He cut deep into the skin, through tendon and muscle, with power and precision. He sometimes came home with his all-white work uniform splattered with dark-red pig blood. It smelt like off roast pork. He looked like an axe-murderer, but was as friendly—in substance and style—as Crocodile Dundee.

He was muscular, tattooed, gentle, hard working, insular, and, at times, inconsolably angry at the world.

'The conscious mind may be compared to a fountain playing in the sun and falling back into the great subterranean pool of subconscious from which it rises,' wrote the Austrian neurologist Sigmund Freud in his book *The Interpretation of Dreams*, published in 1900. He would go on to say:

> Illusions commend themselves to us because they save us pain and allow us to enjoy pleasure instead. We must therefore accept it without complaint when they sometimes collide with a bit of reality against which they are dashed to pieces.

Drawing on the work of eighteenth-century German romantic philosophers, enlightenment-era science, Platonic theory, medieval thinkers, and ancient Hindu texts—and after decades of work—Freud gradually pieced together and popularised a theory that there was more to the mind and to what makes us human than that of which we are consciously aware. Freud believed that there is an unconscious part of the mind that contains our instincts, and thus many of our behaviours, thoughts, and feelings cannot be consciously controlled. Freud saw this part of the mind as also containing memories that had been forgotten but could be recalled, and a place that stored socially unacceptable wishes and desires, trauma, and pain.

Around 1910, Freud's student—the debonair Swiss psychiatrist and psychotherapist Carl Jung—added another layer to Freud's theory of the mind: the idea of the collective unconscious. For Jung, the collective unconscious is not formed by experience, but inherited. This universal, human psychic structure, Jung said, is much like Freud's notion of 'instincts', but it exists in a series of archetypes, symbols, and myths. These innate projections, this readiness to perceive certain archetypal patterns and symbols, is why, according to Jung, children fantasise so much: because they haven't had enough experience to temper their connection to this metaphysical world. Jung believed there were certain archetypal events: marriage, initiation, birth, death, and the separation from parents. He also believed there were archetypal figures — hero, trickster, great mother, great father, child, and devil — as well as archetypal motifs such as deluge, creation, and the apocalypse.

Jung believed it was our culture, history, and personal context that shape these archetypes, thereby giving them their particular shape and form. He also described something called 'The Shadow', which can be both a repressed aspect of ourselves that we don't like or can't deal with, or, in some cases, the entirety of our unconscious mind.

Take it or leave it. Indeed, many leave it, and don't buy into Jung's notion of the collective unconscious, although it's an interesting lens through which to view what I am about to tell you.

'It's fourteen-hundred hours, the subject is inside, all men in their positions, on the ready for when I say "attack",' the general said over a CB radio, from inside his station wagon. He wasn't in uniform, but he was a military man nonetheless, with a rugged face. 'I'll stay put, out the front. You men wait around the corner.'

The general's troops were in cars, strategically scattered around the house of Cassie, a 19-year-old philosophy student. She lived in a wooden Belgrave Heights shack, amid giant mountain gums, and cottages with wind chimes that were — on this grey July day in 1999 — deadly still.

If you flew a helicopter low over the area, you would see Cassie's tin roof, the general's station wagon parked out of the front, another car across the road, two at either end of the street, two behind the property adjoining, and half a dozen others in various strategic exit points in the neighbourhood. They were utes, mainly. All were linked up with a radio, and some were so eager for the attack on 'The Subject' they were revving their cars in excitement. Some had guns for backup, though this would probably be unnecessary. These were big blokes who played football; a couple of them had military training.

'I wanna get him now, boss,' one said, slapping his hand on the steering wheel. 'Can't we just run on in there?'

'Don't worry,' the general said. 'His time will come; he will feel the pain. We just need to be patient, strategic—wait for him to fall into the trap.'

Cassie had been the one to call them in. The 'Subject' was her guest. The 'Subject' was, in fact, me. There was nothing I could do, sitting in Cassie's lounge room amid her art-history and feminism books, on a still, grim mountain day, waiting, just waiting—knowing all the cars were building up outside.

Cassie had misinterpreted a story I had told her the night before: although I was gay, when I was six I had experimented sexually with my 7-year-old female next-door neighbour. Cassie was incredulous, explaining to me—partly through her mad-cutlery eyes, pupils swimming like furious teacups on little spinning plates—the high number of girls who were sexually assaulted in their most vulnerable years, and that men like me were the ones responsible for it.

You should have seen her face that day: with its furious expression, and her long, messy pink hair, she looked like a homicidal troll doll. Although she was having doubts about whether to go ahead with the murder—she looked unsure and guilty—in the end she concluded: 'You have to feel the pain.'

And again: 'You have to feel the pain.'

My God, she must have said it a dozen times over.

And then, when I picked up the phone to call my parents, she took the receiver out of my hand and said, 'That's not a good idea, Luke.'

I was just waiting and waiting for one of the men to burst through the door.

*Kill yourself, Luke, do it. Kill yourself, it's the only way out*, I began to think.

At one stage, she disappeared into the bedroom. I was lying on a mattress in the lounge room, staring up at the layer upon layer of clouds through the windows. There was a strange haze floating in the winter afternoon as the mist set in, and I was struck with a sudden feeling of déjà vu. I felt as defenceless and uncertain as if I were in a dream, my darkest intuitions and fantasies about the world materialising.

I picked up the biggest knife from the kitchen I could find. I walked to the toilet, and locked the door. I pulled the knife across my wrist with full force. It burned, hurting more than I anticipated, like stabbing myself with twenty pins at once. I removed the knife—shit! It had left only the slightest graze. Cassie's big cooking knife was as blunt as a broom handle, and hadn't left a single drop of blood.

Seeing Cassie reappear, I dashed out the back door, slippery as a cat, ducking for cover between her and her housemate's cars as I moved down the driveway. I was heading for my parents' house, about a four-hour walk away.

I passed daffodils and oak trees, and made my way to the bottom of the driveway. The general was no longer there. WTF? *Run, run.*

I snuck around Cassie's car and popped my head over the bonnet to catch a glimpse. Where were they?

I ran up a little-known mud footpath that went between two properties. But they must have somehow realised that I was leaving, because when I got around the corner, there were two utes parked on the street. I tried to make my way through the most deceiving, most rarely used, residential street. But somehow they knew I was going that way. I noticed a panel van parked outside a house. There were more of them. More parked down the next street, and then a few driving down an adjoining road.

*My God*, I thought, *there must be dozens of them*.

It was their military training; they had every corner covered. They had brought together every person who hated me, and every person who *would* hate me if they knew me.

I decided to walk and stay in public until I reached my parents' house. I couldn't think of anybody to call except for the ladies in the local general store. They loved me; we would always have a chat. If I could get in there and ask them if I could hide in there, they could call the police.

The store was on a main road; it was something between a milk bar and a supermarket, dusky and poorly lit, with just three aisles. I went straight to the counter, but there was nobody there, so I hid behind the biscuit display at the end of aisle two.

I waited another five minutes. Where were they? I banged on the back door: 'Please help me, please — they're trying to kill me.' There was no answer. Were these women dead? I had never known that shop to be unattended, let alone for this long. Perhaps they'd also turned on me. Then a panel van turned up out the front, and there was no place to hide. I ran for it.

I ran for five minutes until I reached a house, the last house before the highway, and still a good 15-kilometre walk to my parent's house. It was a highway full of mysterious rolling hills, rickety, dry, rough bushland, kangaroo road-kill, Victoria's second-biggest reservoir (which was fenced off by barbed wire and surrounded by pine trees), and empty farms. It was a highway that usually roared with yobbos and rednecks, and was, on that day, filled with hundreds of cars from the military-trained gang.

I banged on the door, screaming for them to help me, screaming that I needed to call the police. There was no answer, and this was, I concluded, because they were dead. By now, word had spread around the region, and thousands of men were excited by the prospect of my slow, violent, well-deserved death, and they all wanted to join in. Every car along the highway was part of the gang, and even though none had stopped, they were driving past because they were gathering around the next corner. One would eventually stop, I was sure, and drag me in.

At first the road was straight and narrow, and then I turned left onto a road that wound through desolate hills. I walked to the rhythm of stones crunching under my foot, waiting to meet the void and the masters of the void. One kilometre … two kilometres … three … I could feel the impervious rhythm of nature … four kilometres, and I was like the antelope chased by lions, or the witch burned at the stake. The mob continued to drive past, thundering past at 120 kilometres per hour with little restraint. They were driving straight from the heart; they were doing the right thing; I had to feel the pain. This was a finite road with a finite destination. I started wheezing. Five kilometres now, and what's three hours when soon there will be no time left at all?

By now it had become a dark winter's night. I was walking past the reservoir when a car pulled up behind me.

*They have been tormenting me all this time*, I thought.

A girl's voice came from the car.

'Hey Luke, wanna lift?'

It was a girl from high school.

I got in the car: 'Jesus Christ, Claire, fucking help me. Thank God. Drive. Look out—bullets.'

'Um, Luke, are you on drugs?'

'Yes, I had some speed last night, but that's not important. Just drive, drive.'

She drove me to my parents' house. I was screaming at them that people were trying to kill me.

'Cars!' I said. 'All the cars down Wellington Road, they're all part of the gang.'

'But how do you know they weren't just cars on the road?' Mum asked, leaning into me with a meaningful look

Oh.

Oh my.

Right.

I then went on to talk about the 'speed' I had taken the night before.

Oh dear. Revelation — I shouldn't have done that either.

I'd had some kind of episode. And now my parents knew I took drugs, and that I had had a psychotic episode and, fuck, how embarrassing.

I rang Cassie, who was extremely upset. 'How could you have just walked out on me like that, after everything we talked about—'

'What did we talk about?' I asked.

'I was telling you for hours about how sensitive I am to rejection,' she said. 'You just sat there, and then repeated the same question over and over again.'

'What question was that?'

'Is the door green? You wouldn't stop asking me whether the door was green.'

I asked my mum to ring a doctor so I could take some Valium, but she said, 'I think you've taken enough drugs for one night, don't you?'

The next day she took me to a drug counsellor, who said the experience was probably the result of smoking cannabis and using amphetamines. She called the psych ward, who told her they didn't need to come. I told her she was young, stupid, and unhelpful, and left after five minutes.

When I got home, I rang Beck, who immediately passed me to the perfect counsel — her new jailbird boyfriend, Nick, who had a minor history of drug-induced psychosis himself.

I told him the story.

'Brother, there's one thing I've always noticed about you. You watch way too-fucking-many movies' he said, before ascending into a deep, wheezy laugh. 'Even your nut-job fantasies are as unimaginative as some bad Hollywood thriller.'

Touché, Nicholas, touché.

There are two things I know now that nobody told me at the time. First, I had experienced a drug-induced psychosis. Second, I hadn't actually taken 'speed'—I had been taking meth instead.

As we have seen in Chapter 3, from around 1996, drug cooks—and soon many others—discovered that they could make much stronger gear using pseudoephedrine from cold-and-flu tablets; they had runners working for them, who would go from chemist to chemist to buy multiple packets. By adding pseudoephedrine to the process, these cooks were making powdered methamphetamine, and not amphetamine sulphate. While there is no evidence that any crystal meth was being made here (unlike in the US) Rebecca McKetin from ANU has told me that, 'By 1999, in most states, over 95 per cent of amphetamine powder seized when people were arrested for possession and trafficking was actually meth.'

Bit by bit, meth—coming in from China, Thailand, Myanmar, and the Philippines via the post, hidden in footbaths and kids toys—was superseding heroin. Bikies here were upping the ante, and making stronger formulas. This all means that when I first starting taking 'speed' in 1998, it is highly likely that I was among the first few thousand people in Australia to take meth. This is probably because after high school I gravitated toward a group of intravenous drug users, who are usually the first in the chain to get the latest drugs.

So it's fair to say—for whatever reason—that my dream of becoming a reclusive, intellectual psychologist hadn't come to fruition by the time I was nineteen. In fact, perhaps it never was my destiny to be a therapist—I mean, I can't imagine too many people wanting to discuss their problems with somebody whose only advice is 'Please tell the general to go easy on me'.

Dreams still fascinate me, however, and there are three that I have had over and over since I was a teenager.

The first is the feeling of first looking at something, then being curious about it, and then being stuck inside it (like, say, watching a television and then being trapped in it). I find I am in an extremely confined space, and I know that I am going to be stuck there—in terrifyingly cramped contortions—until I die. A psychiatrist told me this likely represented birth trauma; my mum *did* tell me that she had an extremely long, difficult labour, and that I wasn't too happy about having to face the world.

The second recurring dream is that I am on some kind of building structure that seems to move around and change. When I look around, I realise I am on the top of something and at risk of falling off. I try to hang on, but the structure keeps changing shape. I eventually get exhausted trying to hang on, and decide to let myself fall. I enjoy the exhilaration of falling, though I know I will die when I hit the ground, and I always wake up just before I do.

The third and most common recurring dream is one where I am back in the Emerald house I lived in as a teenager, and I am trying to work out what has happened to all the bush in our backyard, and trying to work out ways to replace it, or let it grow back.

Let me provide a bit of context here: while we were living in a small timber house in a neighbouring town, my dad took over managing the piggery he had worked in most of his adult life. The amount of money coming into our household grew exponentially, and so we moved to a big house, twice the size of the old one, on four acres. It was 30 square metres, and looked even bigger because it was thin and long. It had a white roof, colonial windows, three living areas, and four bedrooms. There were floral curtains in nearly every room. The place was heavily alarmed, and every room had movement sensors in it. The house sat half-way up a big hill; for Dad, it was also an entire world away from his childhood of roasted rats, empty stomachs, beatings, grime, and the disempowering shame that went along with those things. Dad used to be so ashamed of his origins that, one day, when one of Mum's friends was coming over with her husband, who worked in a bank, Dad wanted to leave the house. He was worried the man would think he was stupid because he worked in an abattoir. He had eventually taught himself how to read, and Mum had taught him how to write. Now he was managing director of his own business — they'd turned the business around, and now made millions of dollars in revenue.

The new house was surrounded by a ratty collection of grasses, ferns, banksias, and little bush-plants that grew white flowers. It certainly wasn't the lush, wet rainforest. From a distance it was a mess, but when I walked Daisy through it, it was surprisingly diverse, with lots of interesting nooks and crannies. It was so dense you couldn't see far ahead of you, and it gave the impression that the yard went on forever when we sat down among it.

Scared by how close the Ash Wednesday bushfires had come to our first house, Mum and Dad went quickly to work, and got the local fire brigade to burn off all the undergrowth on the property. Mum also regarded the undergrowth as 'untidy'. I didn't want my parents to burn down the scrub, though. I knew — for instance — that it was full of lizards, and 13-year-old me felt particularly sad that they would all fry to death just before Christmas.

I have since had hundreds of dreams about attempting to replant this space. In some dreams, even the remaining eucalypts were gone and replaced by pine trees, with barren ground; in others, everything had been levelled by modest and monotonous portable classrooms. Something had been destroyed and not allowed to grow back; other things weren't allowed to grow at all, or looked unnatural in that setting. In my dreams, I had all sorts of ideas—and subsequent regrets—about setting it all right again. Other times I have that dream, the entire house has been overgrown by the bush, but I am no longer living there. The people inside look at me with confused horror; I am wondering why I never left.

Just before we moved into this house, my parents sent me to a (relatively cheap) private Christian high school, instead of to the local public school in Emerald. I was always getting into trouble there, mainly for not doing any work and for yelling at the teachers. I failed every single subject except phys. ed. in Year 8. We had some strict, old-fashioned teachers at that school—one in particular never let us utter a single word in class. One day, with a water balloon in hand, I walked into a class he was teaching, threw it into the fan, and then ran down the hall, giggling ecstatically. Another day I stood up and told our keyboarding teacher she was a 'stupid fucking bitch'. I was eventually expelled in Year 9 after—on the way to a school camp, and in the middle of nowhere—I stole a bunch of chocolate Big Ms and threw them at a house. A teacher saw me, and as I was already on my last legs there, I was expelled. I was then sent to the local public school.

During my time at the private school, I had tried to climb the social ladder and break in with the popular boys. They were at first a bit iffy with me, and I didn't always get invited to parties. At one party I went to, though, I got really drunk—I was soon able to outdrink most people—and did all sorts of silly things, such as putting baked-beans tins in the fire, and squirting people with tomato-sauce bottles. From then on, I was in.

I am not sure why I was such a little shit when I was that age. I really just wanted to entertain myself and make people laugh.

My school counsellor said it was a combination of 'boredom and low self-esteem'. My mum said I 'lacked self-control'. Indeed, the 'self' was all-important to my family back then — my parents thrived in the new capitalism. Appearance was reality back then, and reality was composed of what we imagined others might be thinking of us.

Mum said she remembers going for drives, away from her alcoholic, abusive household in housing-commission East Malvern, to the big houses around Chadstone Shopping Centre, and daydreaming about how elegant, proper, and peaceful life must have been inside them. She loved the new house; when we moved in, she didn't really need to work. She never really cooked, and we had a cleaner. She spent ten to sixteen hours a day on the computer, playing solitaire. We had no family get-togethers, no traditions, not even a bookshelf; we each had our lounge area, and we never ate dinner together. I no longer had neighbours to run around with. But I did get an expensive tutor who my parents spent thousands of dollars on and many hours driving me into the inner suburb of Camberwell to see each week. This woman — Gillian — was a massive help, without a doubt, and introduced me to books and ideas and writing. She was a psychologist, too, just like I wanted to be.

Mum was often very upset by the things I did. For example, one day she asked me to make her coffee after I got home from school and I said no, because she hadn't been doing anything all day. The next day she told me that I was a horrible person and that this made her cry; she looked at me as if I had thrown her out on the street with no money and nowhere to go. She cried a lot back then. She cried when she and Dad went through months without speaking. She cried for months on end when we found Daisy on the back porch, her jaw in an awkward position, having died of old age when we weren't home.

After the bushes were burnt down, I could see the portable

classrooms of my new school from the back fence. From my lounge room, I could see my classmates waiting for home group in the morning. They were hard to miss—they all had bright-red windcheaters on, which we had to wear with blue trousers and Blundstone boots.

This was the school that was preparing tomorrow's labourers, tradies, and small-time crims—'access to excellence' was its motto.

My 'friends' were always quick to acknowledge my presence once I got over the fence.

'Luke the disgusting faggot is here.'

'Poofter, poofter, cock-sucker,' and so on.

Every morning for three years.

This was the dawn of a new era in my life—I would know now what it was like to be the lowest-ranking male. To use the metaphor of a diseased tree, the problem was that I was blossoming into an adult that some considered to be threatening to the population; an adult that needed to be cut down, turned into sawdust, and buried in a hole to ensure it didn't spread weakness, perversion, and infection. I am, in fact, talking here about the life of a gay teenager in post-AIDS 1990s country Australia.

Mind you, I didn't even see myself as being gay at the time. The trouble had its origins in grade five, before anybody knew what gay was. I had earned a reputation for being able to make guys ejaculate using my hands. Every second guy in my grade was shown this magic trick. Years later, when we all figured what this meant, not a single person came and patted my back in the gym change-rooms and said, 'You gave good hand jobs for one so young, do you want to come to a party on Saturday night?' Rather, it was seen as transgressive and abject—an act of faggotry—and suddenly, like magic, I had no friends: a dangerous proposition at a working-class bush school, where boys liked to start wars.

'Hi, Luke' wasn't something I heard very much in those formative years: the years in which it's generally considered healthy and necessary for a person to have a peer group, which is the first step in a natural and incremental flight from the nest. But I did hear plenty of other things, in high-pitched whiny voices from the grotty little shits at our nondescript public school filled with eucalypts, portable classrooms, and the petty criminals of tomorrow. Every lunchtime and recess I heard myself called a 'cock-licker', a 'poo-pusher', a 'girly-boy', and a 'faggot' because I ran on my toes. For the sake of variety, a group of boys would often call 'poof-poof-poof' to emulate the sound of a chicken as I walked—quite ingenious, really, and quite remarkable the extent of cruelty's entertainment value. Perhaps more amazing was how many derogatory words there were for a boy who liked boys—and how just one of these words could leave the target feeling utterly isolated and defenceless

Here are some of the other highlights:

One morning in Year 9, I found my two best friends amid the sea of red jumpers and the rotten, salty scent of cheap canteen noodles. I had known Leigh and Todd for six years by this stage. They had come to every one of my birthdays, and me theirs. They were an old reliable pair—smart and sensible without being stuffy, low maintenance, and generally pretty easy company. On this morning, they were both sitting in silence, staring ahead, when I put my pencil case down next to one of Leigh's. Without raising his eyes to look at me, Leigh knocked my case to the floor. When I went to put the pencil case back on the table, he picked it up and threw it across the room. A few snickers echoed around the room—though, for the most part, nobody really seemed to be paying attention.

'Don't sit next to us, poofter,' Todd said. When I picked up my pencil case and placed it next to a group of boys down the other end, they said, 'Yeah, don't sit next to us either', and my pencil case once again made its way to the floor.

Once the 'populars' deserted me, the middle-ranking males joined, then the lower-ranking boys, and finally even the lower-ranking girls joined in, on occasion, with choice impersonations of my voice taken straight out of 1980s Hollywood depictions of limp-wristed, constantly horny gays.

One day, I was standing in line during phys. ed. when I felt a thud on my back. I turned around to see the offending basketball bouncing away, and a kid with muscular dystrophy explaining, 'I fucking hate faggots'. I stood there confused, shocked, and horrified as I saw the boy, barely able to stand up from his neurological condition, looking at me as if I was the biggest turd nature had ever produced.

There was one particular group of no less than 15 strapping young lads who lived on farms in the backend district who loved to torment me, and at least half a dozen smaller packs who joined in. I was not only without allies—I was a late bloomer, one of the smallest in my year level by height and frame. Defence was futile, attack was unthinkable, and dobbing them in would have just made it worse.

Seeking even greater thrills, their attacks became more theatrical. Sneak attacks were the favourite. One day, I was standing outside a classroom when I felt a strong push in the back, and 'thud'—I went straight into a metal pole upholding the corrugated-iron roof. I turned around to see a little bully henchman with spiky, light-brown hair and a small neck, his glowing grin slowly becoming a light cackle.

'Look at how red his face gets! Fuck, I could do this every day, just to see how red your faggot face gets,' the henchman said.

Funny indeed. The fact that I had red hair, glasses, braces, and acne—the fact that I was one ugly little bastard—probably just added to the comedic display. Unsurprisingly, those watching laughed raucously; others not privy to the group tried not to laugh, but couldn't help cracking a smile. These were human kids tormenting a disgusting little insect caught in a jar, fascinated by the reactions to their own cruelty. Had it not been me getting thrown into metal poles, perhaps even I would have quietly cracked a smile about how ridiculous it all looked; helpless creatures can react in quite spectacularly pathetic ways when they are attacked.

Teachers often loved the spectacle as well. I never got along well with teachers—though I was often scared to say 'boo' at the new school, when I did act up, I made sure it hit its mark, and the teachers responded with even greater force. One day, I was taken into an office where three middle-aged male teachers took turns in telling me what an awful student I was. I had accused one teacher of being negligent, and refused another when she told me to stop scratching my nuts in class. One told me I would be better off leaving school 'because your work is so crap', and another said, 'I would say most of the staff room hates you, and if I was ask three-quarters of the people in your level, they would say the same thing. Yet you sit here, high and mighty and sanctimonious, like you never do anything wrong.' This went on for about half an hour until tears fell down my cheeks, and the three sat around me, glowing with self-satisfaction at how, despite my 'big mouth', I now didn't 'have anything to say'. About six months after this, I'd left my school bag in a classroom and when I went back to retrieve it, the male teacher whispered under his breath, and then said very sarcastically, 'Sorry, I'm homophobic', at which a group of students broke out in hearty laughter. The same teacher had taught me English in Year 9, and announced halfway through the term, 'It doesn't matter how your good work is, I am not giving you an A.'

There comes a point when you must draw on your reserves to get through things.

Remembering what a war-hungry little shit I was, I decided that I could wage war without any close allies. Why not? I had nothing to lose.

Then came my idea. I listed the seven people who had picked on me the most, and asked people to sign a petition that said, 'If you don't like X, Y, and Z, please sign here and give your reason.' The petition was my attempt to not only enlist a few allies, but to also shame the perpetrators. I had managed to collect dirt on all seven of them over the years—girls who had rejected them, abusive fathers, physical deformities, etc.—all of which were stated on the petition. I collected 80 signatures, and I put copies all over the school. When three of them saw me with a couple of surveys, they snatched them out of my hand. The no-neck henchman said, 'We've got the muscle-power and the evidence—you're fucked.' The second he finished his sentence, I punched him straight in the face. The other two joined in to help him, and kept throwing punches. After about thirty seconds, a teacher came over and broke it up.

By this stage, I was growing into my body, and doing athletics training nearly every day. I became enraged, yelling that they had 'shit for brains', and that it would take 'less than an hour to get another 80 signatures' and that they 'should just mind their own fucking business from now on'. The bullies were incredulous; they rang me at home threatening to stab me, and lined up along my fence. I shouted, 'There's fuck-all you can do about it—I have 80 people backing me up now.'

A week after everything died down, thanks to some stern words from the school headmaster, I got another phone call: 'I'm one of those guys you've been writing all that shit about. You're not going to get away with this. You better watch your back; you won't get away with this. One day, one day, maybe years and years after school, there'll be a massive gang of us, and we'll get you and your family, too,' he said.

But I *had* gotten away with it. Despite this victory, I left school, and finished it by correspondence. Academic and sporting achievements followed. I had my first real group of friends in a long while. I officially came out as gay.

Although my parents responded reasonably well to my coming out—both said they didn't really mind—my relationship with them was becoming increasingly difficult. They told me they didn't want to think about me having sex. Dad said he thought it was just a phase. I had only ever heard him mention gay people twice; both times were to say that they 'made him sick'. When I caught crabs, Mum yelled at me about having a responsible sex life. Dad wanted me to move out. My sister had already moved out, and was estranged from the family after a bad fight with Mum.

Mum had particular difficulties with the fact that I now dressed in op-shop clothes and had friends. She would call me when I was at a friend's house, crying and demanding I come home. When I came home, I had to take off my op-shop clothes and dress myself in the surf clothes I used to wear when I was fourteen. Eventually, she said I wasn't allowed to dress in the clothes I'd bought for myself in the house, and I had to keep them at a friend's place.

One terrible fight led to my mum throwing me out of the house. I hadn't finished Year 12 at the time. I had nowhere to stay and no money. I begged a friend to let me stay with him, and I stole all my food. Determined to survive with flair, I dressed up as a 'person with a disability'—complete with neck brace and op-shop clothes—stole a raffle book, and went door-knocking, asking for money for the 'U/21 disabled hockey team to compete in the upcoming national championships in Canberra'.

By this stage, while I was selling stolen raffle tickets in order to eat, my parents had taken advantage of a new tax-incentive scheme called negative gearing, and now owned three properties. Then I got a call from my tutor who told me, 'Your mother is not well at the moment. She needs to go the doctor and get herself put on medication. You probably need to stay away until she gets better.'

After a couple of weeks, my mum rang and apologised, and I moved back home. I kept going with Year 12, but then halfway through—out of nowhere—things started to change. I felt tired, unmotivated, and sulky. I didn't want to leave the house. I felt a strange sense of dread and disaster every time I did go out. I had started spending time with a group of gay guys who lived in Prahran, but over time I found them more and more confident, good-looking, and intimidating, and eventually I cut my ties with them. Once I got my marks halfway through the year, I realised they would be enough to get me into an Arts degree at La Trobe University, and after that I did the bare minimum, including during exams, where I walked out after the minimum one-hour time.

Often, the onset for serious mental illness—such as bipolar disorder or schizophrenia—occurs at about the age of seventeen or eighteen. Until then, the individual might be weird, or misbehaved, or withdrawn, or normal. My uncle Gary didn't develop schizophrenia until he experienced acute work stress at the age of thirty-five. But when he was seventeen, he spent a period of about two years hardly speaking, not socialising, and just sitting in his room. It was possible I had caught the family disease. I had certainly caught one sort of family disease—an obsession with appearances. Every time I saw myself in the mirror, I saw nothing but the world's ugliest person, and assumed that everybody saw the same—and then they saw a faggot.

By the time I finished high school, I had trouble leaving my room under any circumstances. When I did, high-pitched alarms went off inside my head, and a prickly little echidna spun around slowly in my stomach. I was at the point of having to drum up the courage even to go my local shopping centre. Once I walked through the bushland next to my house to the bus stop across the road. I took a deep breath that soon turned into rushed panting, and walked back through the bushland and into my house, where I didn't leave my room for another couple of weeks. I was spooked by the slightest noise. I watched TV all day, and smoked in my room. I read *Smash Hits* magazine, and spent hours with my headphones on, imagining I was a pop star — as if I were thirteen again.

A few months later, I started my philosophy degree at La Trobe, in Melbourne's outer-northern suburbs. I missed the first two weeks of the course because of 'my friend, the echidna'. When I finally made it to campus, I left a lecture to hide in the toilets for a good hour, before catching the bus and going back home. My room became both a refuge and a scene of minor carnage. I shaved uneven patches out of my hair and dyed it green. I started cutting myself with a kitchen knife, and, at one stage, I had three piercings under my lip.

Eventually, I met the town's hippies with their makeshift homes, their tepees, and was introduced to their magic herbs, tea-tree cleaning products, and all-night Shamanic shindigs in the bush. I adored their healthy eating, near-asexuality, and earthy liberalism. A few of the women invited me along to my first-ever rave. These events, held deep in the forest, were a wonderful mixture of counter-culture, individualism, and archetypal tribalism — I felt as if I had found my tribe. I do wonder now if I would have liked it so much were it not for the drugs — at my first rave, I tried my first ecstasy. So while I salvaged the year and managed to get out of my room, there was a caveat on my newfound freedom: I couldn't go out without first taking so much ecstasy that I lost sense of who I was and where I was going.

I tried 'speed' one night in mid-1998, when we couldn't get any E. I didn't get as 'off chops' on the white powder, but I rather liked the fact that it gave me confidence without turning me into a blubbering mess. Many of my friends used syringes, which seemed exciting and edgy. I was very curious, but the hippie women were reluctant to show me how to do it because they said I had 'addictive tendencies'. However, after a few months of my nagging, they gave me my first intravenous shot of amphetamines in a glittery station wagon — which the owner called her 'unicorn' — outside a converted mansion nightclub in St Kilda.

So I guess it went like this: the amphetamines gave me confidence and, even more than that, a window into an idealised, transcendental reality — which, for all I thought at the time, was actually a mystical *parallel* reality. At the start of 1999, just before my nineteenth birthday, I popped the ecstasy pill to end all ecstasy pills at an outdoor bush doof at a place inappropriately named Mount Disappointment. The world took on a wonderfully cartoonish flavour as I thought, *This is how I always wanted life to be.* This led me on a voyage to rediscover that high, and when other ecstasy pills didn't do the trick, I turned again to needles. I claimed study allowance from Centrelink — even though I never went to uni — and with the proceeds I pumped my veins full of 'speed': monthly, then weekly, then during the week. I eventually stopped going out to raves and dance parties, and just stayed home and took drugs instead. This went on for a good twelve months; I was a 'pleasure glutton', besotted by the broom that swept all the dread away. It was like alchemy, like magic — who wouldn't want that?

According to Jung, one of the most universal and universally misunderstood archetypes is Mercurius — aka the Roman god, Mercury — known for his speed and mobility. In the ancient art of alchemy, the Earth's three principle substances were mercury, sulphur, and salt—in fact, the Sanskrit word for alchemy is *Rasavātam,* which means 'the way of mercury'. Jung saw Mercurius as the essence of the unconscious. He also believed that Mercurius was the 'trickster' archetype—a shape-shifter who could change gender and meanings, who was ambiguous, paradoxical, and duplicitous. A destroyer, Mercurius is also volatile, meaningful, and difficult to contain. According to Jung, it is only through Mercurius that we can see the fullness of our psyche, including evil.

The more I injected 'speed', the more the meanings of things started to change and to take on a sinister turn. I would be having a rapid-fire conversation with someone, and everything they said would sound as if it had a deliberate, sly, tricky, persecutory double meaning. Language, at times, totally disintegrated. I would take odd words out of somebody's sentences when they were talking, and I would think they were directed at me. Somebody might mention 'underwear', and I would think they had caught me masturbating. Or somebody would be talking about a guy they hated called 'Pete', and I would think they were passive-aggressively telling me in code what they hated about me. Most of the time I would be able to find my way in the conversation and realise I was being paranoid. But then came a day, after a year or more of building up, when I couldn't snap out of it at Cassie's—where it felt as if the apocalypse had come. Mercurius was, perhaps, riding around with me that day. In doing so, it revealed a painful, dark shadow.

After my psychotic breakdown, the clouds seemed to clear—it was as if a cyst had been burst open, and I could start to live again. The anxiety eased. I went back to uni. The shadow had come into light. The psychosis had proved a creative starting point. Things were starting to change—both for me, and in another part of the world ...

In the rugged, remote, wildlife-rich mountains covering

a corner of Burma (now Myanmar), Laos, and Thailand, the monsoon rains hadn't come for three years. Amid the hills was an area that was more or less controlled by a renegade ethnic gathering called the United Wa State Army. The military wing of a fringe Burmese political group formed after the collapse of the Burmese Communist Party in 1989, the army took control of the land bordering Thailand, as well as the region's opium poppy fields. In 1997, South-East Asia still accounted for well over half of the world's opium production. As the new millennium came, the drought was broken, and was followed by abnormal flooding and frost in Burma.

It would prove to be the drought before the storm in more ways that one. Drugs were the main source of the army's income, and they began searching for alternatives.

# Chapter Five

# Rise and fall

BECK, AGE NINETEEN, gave birth during Melbourne's spectacularly hot, fire-ridden summer of 1998. A beautiful rosy-cheeked, hot-tempered child, Hayley was born at the Ferntree Gully Hospital on 11 February, and returned with her mother about a week later to a rented, non-air-conditioned share house in Rowville in Melbourne's flat, sprawling south-east suburbs.

Many of Beck's adolescent tendencies had continued into adulthood. If somebody in town believed in ghosts, or had a bad deformity, or had spent most of their life in jail, you could rest assured that Beck would track them down and be knocking on their door with a bottle of goon, ready to entertain.

Along her travels, she got to know one man named Barry, a former television-station electrician who'd hurt himself at work and then became lost in his own mind and its many theories—including one that Easter eggs were actually grenades wrapped in foil. Barry, in turn, introduced Beck to Nick while she was pregnant. He was a tall, muscular, kind-of-French-looking, handsome lad. Aged twenty-seven when they met, Nick hadn't spent a single birthday out of prison in his entire adult life. He was a big fellow, but not usually a violent one. In fact, Nick was a bit of an intellectual; he read Dostoyevsky and maths textbooks when he was in prison, and took classes in physics. When he was out of prison, he stole at every opportunity. His main trade was robbing houses, but he also robbed service stations — sometimes with a weapon (although his physical presence was often enough to get the attendant to cooperate) — when he got desperate.

Nick and Beck got together, and he moved into the Rowville house when Beck was six months pregnant. When she entered the late stages of her pregnancy, he would come home after a busy day with new toys, prams, and electronic goods. Beck was always uncomfortable with stealing, though no man had ever lavished her with such gifts. She told me she often felt terribly guilty knowing that somebody came home to find their baby's goods missing.

Home robberies became at least a weekly event for Nick and some of his friends — 'rorts', they called them. They often sold the goods at second-hand stores, or traded them for pot, acid, and ecstasy.

On one occasion, when Nick and his friend Jason had cased at least a dozen homes in one particular area of Rowville and had made their way out the side window of a house with a few watches, phones, and entertainment consoles, they noticed a police car gliding toward them as they made their escape in their car. The police sirens screeched and their lights flashed, and Jason hit the accelerator. A chase ensued through the labyrinth of Rowville's monotonous terracotta-roofed suburbia, and when they got to the first traffic lights, the police instructed them through a loudspeaker to pull over and surrender; instead, Jason revved the car, and reversed into the front of the police car, over and over, in an attempt to blow up its engine.

Police cars are built to withstand such force, however, and the chase continued into neighbouring Lysterfield. At the next traffic lights, a panicked Jason — young and thus far without a criminal record—gave himself up. Nick made a run for it, until the police found him about to get on a bus a kilometre away.

Nick was charged and sentenced to around ten months in jail, which he didn't mind; he always said he preferred life on the inside.

Beck's other housemates had also moved out, and so at this stage, when Hayley was about ten months old, she asked me to move in to help out. So I did.

I had been scared of Hayley until she was seven months old. I was scared of breaking her. I didn't know how to act around a creature who I thought I was supposed to bond with, and for the first part of her life, my presence was neither here nor there. Then one day, when Hayley was a rosy-cheeked, sweet-smelling 8-month-old sitting on the lounge room of Beck's parent's lounge room—not long before Beck moved to Queensland—I picked her up. She looked at me with confusion, and then she smiled. The next day I picked her up again and she giggled. Soon thereafter, nearly every time I saw her she held out her arms to me. Before Hayley was born, I had no idea how much we humans need each other, how much we need love and attention.

A few days after I moved in, I noticed Beck was no longer as sulky or needy. She had managed to find rhythm in this new life, had become, in fact, one fearsome bitch.

Beck's mum had been a bank teller and an aged-care worker; her dad was a senior nurse at a big public hospital. While she enjoyed being a budget 'gangsta's moll', it went deeper than that; she also enjoyed the thrill of the fall away from her hardworking family. She found her life relaxing and liberating, even funny. She seemed to almost thrive in it.

A few weeks into this new house set-up, we had a guy named Andrew move in. Andrew was a heroin addict who had tuberculosis and constantly threw up in the kitchen sink. He had also, much to his pride, been to jail and learnt the art of rape threats. One day he threatened the elderly man next door: 'I'll tie up your wife and put a knife to her throat,' he said. Within a week, the house was for sale.

Another day I was sitting in my room, stoned and daydreaming, when Andrew and Beck started arguing. It didn't take long before he started throwing around couches, and, as I sat petrified in my room, I heard him say he was going to rape her 'in your toerag arse' and then screamed that he would track down her younger sisters.

He then said—and I quote—'you toeragin me dowwwll', before threatening her mum, her nanna, and her dad. To this day, we don't know what he meant.

After about a minute's silence, I heard Beck start laughing—at first sincerely, and then deliberately and provocatively loudly—and say, 'First of all, Andrew, I am not a fucking toerag, and second of all *you are going to rape my dad.*'

And that was the end of that: a new era of Beck had begun.

We must have quoted that day a thousand times since, at random times and with the best comic timing we could muster: for example, while waiting in a doctor's surgery she would say, 'Oh shit, I forgot to ask my dad if Andrew has raped him yet'. That and 'dowwwll' would thereafter become permanent parts of our secret lexicon.

Despite the fun we had, I too moved out not long after this incident; this new Beck was constantly screaming and yelling abuse. She herself only stayed in that house for a little while longer before moving to Queensland. Then Nick got out of jail, and moved in with her into a tiny two-bedroom house in a southern suburb of Brisbane.

As for me? Well, after surviving the violent homicidal urges of hordes of angry large men—both real and imaginary—I settled back into uni, post-psychosis, with newfound confidence and a newfound addiction to reading. I took classes such as Classic Literature, Existentialism, Reason and Logic, and Postmodernism. I read obsessively. I avoided drugs, and sought to find the answers to what had happened to me in the materials I was reading. I began living with some of the hippies from Cockatoo in a large Northcote warehouse with a bunch of musicians, painters, and circus performers. We had no bathroom, and there were so many people coming and going all the time that at some stage I learnt how to look people in the eye again. After a semester, I was still at a loss to understand my 'great decline', but I became so involved in the texts it didn't seem to matter. My friends from Cockatoo seemed to get over using drugs as well, and became involved in theatre, painting, and circus.

After a few months, it occurred to me that the house wasn't quite my fit: I had yet to have any experience with gay guys or the gay world. I found a gay housemate online, and moved into a place in Collingwood. He turned out to be a 45-year-old Telstra exec who moped constantly about the loss of his younger ex-boyfriend (and his 'elongated cock') and who also injected 'speed' (powdered meth) on the weekends. I injected with him, and still didn't have the confidence to walk into a gay club. I must have walked up to the door of The Peel a dozen times before walking away again, petrified. I was, quite simply, worried that I wouldn't be attractive enough in a world where looks and sex mean everything.

Other than that, I found the house too clean and too neat. I don't remember much about it except for my housemate's loud middle-aged queeny queens coming over, and don't remember much of that except for the pungent smell of their cologne. I had started to feel lonely by this time—I'd failed to make my way into gay culture, and I was missing Beck and her cavalcade of addicts, gypsies, tramps, and thieves.

One day, on one of our many phone chats—we had stayed in touch—she invited me to go and live with her again, and I took her up on her offer.

I spent a week in King's Cross before going up to Brisbane, where I took a train south to a small town 20 kilometres from Brisbane, in the heart of Logan City. I arrived to find a cute, basic, warm, sunny town with palm trees, plate-sized cane toads, and a large Islander population.

'So I'm in a relationship with a criminal, I'm on the dole, I live in the welfare and crime capital of Queensland on dole street. I'm on the dowwwwll, man. The dowwwwwll,' Beck said as she met me at the train station.

'You make me sick,' I replied.

And so it began.

Beck lived in a tiny house on sand like soil, with a gigantic eucalypt in the backyard. She woke me up every morning at 8.50, tapping on a bong with the lighter and saying in a faux-posh voice:

'Luuuuuuke, Denise is on.'

And so every morning, when Hayley (then two) was in day-care, we would sit in front of the television, ripping down bongs and watching the Denise Drysdale show for two hours, normally so stoned we couldn't follow what was going on. Then the Olympics started, and we took turns making angry, stoned phone calls to Channel 7 about how disrespectful it was to Denise that the program would be off-air for three weeks.

By the time I arrived in that winter of 2000, Beck and Nick were using intravenous 'speed' as well, though not every day (mainly because they couldn't afford to). Beck wasn't showing too many signs of going nutty, and while I *did* use, the big psychotic episode I had in 1999 — and the break from drugs I had taken after it — had seemed to clean out some of my demons. I decided not to inject it, but to snort it instead.

Fortuitously for me, Beck and Nick had made friends with a few gay guys from Brisbane. Brisbane back then was slow and friendly, more like a country town than a city; the high-rises in the CBD felt very artificial because it really *could* have been a country town in Gippsland or Central Victoria. The gay guys were less intimidating: less concerned with the way they dressed, friendlier, and more down-to-earth. The gay clubs felt like country pubs, and for the first time, I found myself going out all the time without feeling much in the way of anxiety.

I began to feel comfortable in my own skin, although life in Woodridge could be a little rough at times. One of our most frequent visitors was a guy named 'Filthy' who was in his mid-sixties and had tattoos all over his face and body. He used to rob houses, and pawn what he'd stolen in second-hand shops. He would come to our house, sit there in the kitchen — bone-thin — with a syringe, and inject himself with powdered meth through a huge track-mark. He would stare into space with his chin moving up and down, just like an old woman's might do involuntarily while she knitted or did the crossword.

We also had regular visits from a woman who lived across the road. She had three young children and a shaved head. One night, she came over asking if she could take some of our blankets or mattresses.

'Ours are all being used, sorry,' I said.

'Well, we have people staying over.'

'Sorry, we need them,' I replied.

'Well, so do we,' she said, staring at me like a serial killer.

Beck then screamed abuse from the bedroom, 'Fuck off, Simone, you stupid bitch, or else I'll come over there and beat the fuck out of you and your skinny runt excuse for a fucking boyfriend.'

Simone remained expressionless, staring at me, while I smiled awkwardly and slowly closed the door in her face.

Another day, I was lying in bed, half-stoned, in the middle of the afternoon, listening to Beck and Nick argue in their bedroom. We'd all had 'speed' — which, of course, was powdered

meth — the night before. I could only half make out what they
arguing about. Then, in an instant, it all boiled over. I heard the
bedroom door fling open.

'Well fucking go then, go, get out!' Beck yelled, her anger
tinged with anguish and fatigue.

I heard him mumble something back, to which she let out a
cross between a scream and a gasp. 'You fucking arsehole! How
could you be so cruel?' This was followed by a loud, hollow
'pop' — like a bottle being shot with a gun — that jolted me right
out of bed. I opened the door to see Beck picking up whatever
she could reach in the kitchen, as Nick rather sheepishly tried to
defend himself from the attack. She was a flurry of wild brown
hair and garbled swear words as she first smashed two coffee cups
over his head, then picked up a large frying-pan.

'Stop it, stop it, please, please,' I said. 'What the fuck is going
on?'

Beck stopped, and Nick stepped out on the balcony.

'He's going to slit Thor's throat,' she said.

'Why?'

'He said he wanted to leave, he said he doesn't love me
anymore, so I asked him what he was going to do with Thor and
he said he was going to slit his throat.'

With that, she started howling and ran into the bedroom;
Hayley was thankfully in day-care. I went outside to the balcony.
Nick had his back to me, and was smoking a rollie. 'Nick,' I said.

'Yep,' he replied, turning around to reveal a spatter of blood
on his forehead that had somehow already dried.

'You are not really going to slash Thor's throat, are you?'

'Well, what else am I supposed to do, she wants me gone.'

'Listen, Nick, I'll look after Thor, Beck will look after Thor,
and if we can't, then someone else will.'

He turned around again, looking across the palm trees and
the dishevelled little houses.

'Nick, Thor is a very nice dog. He is his own being. He deserves to have a full, lovely life and we can all make sure that happens.' At that, Nick put on his backpack and stomped down the steps. 'It's a shame nobody ever gave a living fuck about me,' he said, his anger escalating. He was breathing faster and faster, his body heaving like the Incredible Hulk, until finally he began to scream. He left the house, and walked (and screamed) all the way down the street. He never came back.

By the end of the year, Beck and I had both returned to Melbourne. For a long time after this, we again went our separate ways. But in her world, I had started to grow into myself. I had survived and even thrived around her criminal friends. It gave me confidence, and, no longer crippled with anxiety, I felt it was time to get more involved in life. In Melbourne, however, I found people a little more intimidating, and I had next to no friends by the time I got back. Also, I was nearly twenty-one and had neither been in a relationship nor really even had sex. But the biggest problem, the one that had stayed with me since my drug binges of the late 1990s, was that strange thing I had been unable to articulate—my confusion about what was real, and, in particular, the fact that I kept hearing hidden meaning in people's words. I would be talking to someone, and I would hear a word and believe it was referring to me, or that the other person knew something secret about me, or that they were doing an impersonation of me. I couldn't even explain at the time, but I was—to put it mildly—one drug-fucked fucker.

I picked out a psychologist at random from the Yellow Pages. A week later, I had an appointment at his Clifton Hill terrace house. He was a small man in his seventies, crippled in some way—he had both a limp and shoulders that sat crookedly enough to suggest he may have had a slight hunchback. When I told him about my lack of friends, he went quickly to work through the categories and criteria he had learnt over his many decades of work as a therapist, and suggested that Schizoid Personality Disorder (SPD) possibly summed me up best — but that ultimately I didn't fit the criteria.

(SPD is a personality disorder characterised by a lack of interest in social relationships, and a tendency towards a solitary lifestyle — which could also describe somebody who is introverted or whose confidence has been destroyed by being alienated from society because of the moral taboos of the time.)

When I explained to him that I kept hearing nasty references to myself when I heard people talking, and that I had 'paranoia', he disputed this, saying it wasn't paranoia but 'low-grade depression'. He suggested I take anti-depressants, but I didn't want to because my only experience with them had been negative. But, of course, in retrospect what I was suffering from was low-grade psychosis, and what I needed was a short course of low-dose anti-psychotics.

In the second session, he told me to join groups that fitted my interests if I wanted to make friends. In the third session, he asked to see my penis.

Yes, my psychologist asked to see my penis. Out of the blue, and over and over again.

Needless to say, I left, but eventually I took him up on his suggestion of getting involved in things that interested me, in order to build a life and make friends.

I started volunteering for a gay community-television program, and soon after met my first boyfriend, and another guy whom we moved in with. We started doing a radio show together — twice a week, midnight till 6.00am — on an outer-suburban radio show in Mill Park.

Around the same time, on a warmish, breezy night in the slightly old-fashioned, middle-class, beachside suburb of Moorabbin in the south-east suburbs of Melbourne, just before the start of the new millennium, Neil Mellnor was working his usual phone shift at a drug and alcohol counselling line. After more than twenty years working as a social worker, Mellnor had pretty much seen and heard it all. On that night, he received a call from a woman who earlier that night had been forced to call the police after her daughter's boyfriend had destroyed the house. The police in turn called an ambulance, and paramedics administered drugs to bring the boyfriend under control. Of all the phone calls and clients he had seen over the years, he couldn't remember anybody else who had presented as this distressed and confused. This would be, in fact, Mellnor's first professional encounter with methamphetamine, and it left him with no doubt that something had changed.

'The extremity of the event and the distress involved really stood out for me,' he said. 'The mother was absolutely petrified. What also struck me was that she said the boyfriend—who was coming down at the time—was not usually violent. The reason why I became so fearful of this drug, despite working in the drug and alcohol field for so long, is the way it changed people's character; it seems to make people violent, aggressive, impulsive, and it gives them strength and a sense of purpose that alcohol doesn't.'

After doing some reading, Mellnor realised he was dealing with methamphetamine, and a deluge of similar calls would follow in the coming months.

As Burma's opium fields wilted at the end of the millennium, and were then all but destroyed by the extreme flooding that broke the drought, and the highly abnormal frosts that followed, the Taliban cracked down on opiate production in Afghanistan. At the same time, the Australian Federal Police were given extra resources and began to get a handle on, and thereby reduce, high-level heroin importation networks; a number of key arrests and some major seizures would follow. Around Christmas in 2000,

Australia experienced an unprecedented reduction in the supply of heroin. Unsurprisingly, the price of heroin rose from $218 a gram to $381. Dealers went to work with cutters—the purity of heroin fell from 60 per cent to 20 per cent. The Illicit Drug Reporting System found a continuing drop in the number of fatal heroin overdoses, which went from 345 in 1999–2000 to 265 in 2000–01. This was the period that became known as the 'heroin drought'.

Many people thought that if heroin became more expensive, dealers' profits would increase and heroin users would commit even more crime to fund their habits. What happened instead was that heroin use, and crimes such as theft and robbery, fell like a stone.

The national robbery rate fell 30 per cent; the national burglary (which, unlike robbery, does not involve the use of force) rate fell 50 per cent; and the national motor-vehicle theft rate fell 56 per cent. The New South Wales robbery rate is now back to where it was in the early 1990s, while the burglary and motor vehicle theft rates in New South Wales are lower than they were in 1990.

The absence of heroin didn't mean the nation's chronic drug-injecting population just gave up drugs and started mid-week social tennis, though. The hunger remained; many injectors love the medicinal eroticism of the needle, as well as the ritual of injecting. Australia's intravenous-drug users would go searching for something else to fill the hole. In 2003, a former prison inmate named 'Scotty the Barber' told Radio National's *Background Briefing* that in some cases, he knew users who shot up conventional medicines (that they knew would not give them a high) and even Vegemite. So, taken altogether, it's not really surprising that it didn't take long for Australia's cohort of drug addicts to shift to another white substance, which offered a very different type of buzz—methamphetamine.

—

Dr Sandy Gordon, then head of intelligence for the Australian Federal Police, would tell the Global Economy of Illicit Drugs conference in London on 26 June 2001 that the East Asia-Pacific's economy had grown by 8 per cent in the 1980s and 7 per cent in the 1990s:

> Although there are clear benefits from development, it can also bring harm, especially in the social sphere. In Asia, rapid urbanisation and development increased working hours in the building, transport, and service industries, resulting in major labour market dislocation. Consumption of amphetamines helped workers cope with these longer hours.

Indeed by this stage, methamphetamine had already replaced heroin as the problem drug in Thailand, and crystal meth was the most commonly used drug in the Philippines. Gordon went on to explain that crackdowns on heroin and methamphetamine by authorities in Thailand had created opportunities for crime groups operating in the Golden Triangle:

> Production of amphetamines in Burma was also facilitated by another development, this time in China. With the advent of economic liberalisation in China, many of the inefficient state-run chemical plants lost their captive markets and could not find new ones. This provided an incentive to 'turn a blind eye' to chemical precursor diversion. It is noteworthy that the very routes now used to take heroin out of Burma could also be used in reverse to bring precursors back in.

The 'Burma problem' resulted in China signing an anti-drugs cooperation agreement with ten other Association of Southeast

Asian countries. Intelligence would later reveal that Asian organised-crime gangs targeted war-torn South Pacific nations to manufacture drugs in the hope of targeting Australia. In June 2001, then new AFP chief Mick Keelty told the *Herald Sun* he believed that the heroin shortage may have been a deliberate strategy by crime czars to shift their business to the more profitable methamphetamine, which could be made entirely inside drug factories.

All the signs were pointing in the same direction. A total of 82 kilograms of crystal meth was seized in the 2000–01 year compared with 971 grams in 1997–98; the number of police detainees found with methamphetamine in their system jumped from 10 per cent in 2000 to 31 per cent in 2001. Research from the Illicit Drug Reporting System showed that of the 910 illicit-drug users surveyed in 2000, just 16 per cent named meth as their drug of choice; by 2001, that figure had jumped to 25 per cent. By the end of 2000, *The Sydney Morning Herald* would publish an article saying that 'researchers across Australia have documented an unprecedented rise in the presence and use of methamphetamine, the derivative of amphetamine best known locally as "ice" or "shabu". The numbers, they say, are unexpected and the fear is that it is being manufactured locally, heralding further rises'. Nearby New Zealand witnessed a similar increase in methamphetamine use, with past-year prevalence increasing from 2.9 per cent in 1998 to 5 per cent in 2000.

Throughout 2000–01, the use of methamphetamine among injecting drug-users increased in almost every state and territory. Relaxed and comfortable Australia was speeding up.

The number of clandestine-lab detections in Australia rose from 95 in 1997 to 201 in 2000, and to 240 in 2001. In March 2003, the annual Australian Crime Commission Illicit Drug Data Report found that amphetamine labs had increased fivefold since 1996 to almost 250 in 2002. The report would say that the overwhelming quantities of methamphetamine precursor chemicals that were being imported (ephedrine and pseudoephedrine) were coming in from Chinese and Filipino ports, with Myanmar, China, and India also playing key roles in meth production across the Asia-Pacific region. A few years later, it was thought that Myanmar was the biggest amphetamine producer in the world, though most of its precursor chemicals would come from China. Three hundred and fourteen clandestine labs were detected in 2002–03, gradually rising to 390 in 2005–06.

While Australia's first meth outbreak was making old criminals richer, new criminals rich, and plunging ordinary citizens into the world of crime, others would see their burgeoning criminal careers draw to a close. By 2001, Richard Walsh — the truck-driver turned dealer we met in Chapter 3 — wanted to limit his risk by making sure he was only dealing to and with high-level bikies who he could trust. By now, Walsh was a sergeant-at-arms in the local chapter of the Nomads and one of his customers, a man called Peter Bennett, had been unable to repay a drug debt to Walsh's de facto Julie Clarke. So Walsh agreed to let Bennett work off the debt by running drugs between Queensland and Newcastle. Peter's wife, Wendy, was also employed by the Walsh household as a nanny, cleaner, and tester of amphetamines.

The Nomads lent Bennett a gun to provide him with protection during his inter-state drug runs, but it was seized by police during a search. To punish him for losing the gun, the Nomads beat Bennett so badly he needed hospital treatment. A short time later, Walsh denied Bennett a long-promised Christmas bonus.

By this stage, Bennett was furious and plotted his revenge, deciding to become a police informer in March 2001. His wife also informed, all the while working for Walsh and Clarke. The quality of the information being received led New South Wales police to throw more funding at the operation and the Drug Squad—along with Northern Region police—set up Strike Force Sibret.

On 23 September 2001, Strike Force Sibret made their penultimate move: Walsh's HiLux was stopped near Murwillumbah with a heavy load of drugs—he now had to do the runs himself without Bennett around. At the same time, raids were conducted at thirteen properties in Newcastle, northern New South Wales, and on the Gold Coast; forty-three people, including sixteen Nomads, were charged. Walsh's de facto Julie Clarke also gave evidence against the accused. Among those arrested, charged, and eventually sentenced was Todd Little—the illiterate drug cook who had become rich making his meth formula. Police recovered $1.5 million in stolen vehicles and other items from the Nomads in Newcastle. As for Walsh, he would receive a sentence of thirty-two years—the longest ever given for a non-importation drug offence in Australia. Walsh had been charged with supplying an entire tonne of kilograms, but pleaded guilty to, and was sentenced for, supplying 400 kilograms. Sibret would go down as one of the biggest hits on an outlaw motorcycle gang in Australian history.

In September 2002, a softly spoken 33-year-old, Damien Peters—slim, tattooed, with messy, wavy hair—murdered two male lovers in the house the three of them shared. In a gruesome scene, he cut off one of their heads, before disembowelling them, and flushing their organs down the toilet. Peters had taken meth on the afternoon of the crime, and was also found to be using steroids, methadone, and anti-depressants. Psychiatrist Dr Yvonne Skinner, who examined Peters in preparation for the trial, found no underlying pathology, personality, environmental, or cognitive factors that created a basis for his attack. Instead, Dr Skinner's report concluded that Peters' actions 'did not arise from an underlying condition, but from the transitory effect of the drug "Ice" amphetamine'.

It's unclear from the legal records whether Peters was taking crystallised meth or powdered meth. But the crime occurred just before several major hospitals around the nation — one of which was St Vincent's in Sydney — began reporting daily or near daily incidence of patients presenting with amphetamine psychosis. Perth seemed particularly hard hit, with record seizures at customs; *The West Australian* newspaper would report Graylands hospital being the first to report that ice was wreaking havoc in their emergency room. Although there was increased awareness of these drugs, there was also a misunderstanding about the difference between 'speed' and 'meth'. 'Ice' and 'meth' were used interchangeably when referring to both crystallised and powdered meth, which are very different drugs.

We didn't know it then, but the worst was yet to come.

By 2001, I was working as a glassie at a big nightclub on Chapel Street. This is a time I remember for cleaning up toilet paper and vomit, for the odours of sweaty bodies, cigarette smoke, stale cellar beer, and Scotchguarded carpets, and for thunderous beats that vibrated through my body at six in the morning when all I wanted to do was go home. I was soon involved in Chapel Street's 'hipster' drug scene, and was taking drugs all weekend as I worked. I remember walking outside into the bright spring morning light and sitting in the car, waiting for my friends to come.

This was also a time of important political change: September 11 happened, and then the Afghanistan invasion and the subsequent debate over refugees. At that moment, sitting in the car with no energy and no direction, my life felt frivolous, selfish, and insular. I felt like a stupid, hyperactive kid who hadn't been allowed to go on a rollercoaster, and then, when his parents were out, snuck into the fair and went on the rollercoaster over and over and over again — up/down/vomit/thrilling/surprising/

look-no-hands/up/down/up/down for weeks and weeks and weeks. Eventually, it got, well … boring. After three days of not sleeping, when the thrill was well and truly gone, I stopped to rest. I thought of all the beaches, all the forests, all the things I was missing out on, realising that there was more to life than a joy ride. Aside from anything else, in 2001 it was still more socially acceptable to be homophobic than to be homosexual. My battle scars from high school seemed to have healed, though; I met gay men who had suffered far worse, and I decided now was the time for a second round at bringing down the bigots.

I also felt like a failure career-wise—that I had wasted a few crucial years I could have spent building my resume. I was nearly twenty-two, and working deep into the night sweeping floors and picking up glasses. Many of my peers had graduated uni, and had already started their careers. I had an abiding sense of status anxiety when I started my quest to have a professional, middle-class job—but it was then or never.

We had stopped doing the community radio show, and instead were doing theatre. We had also continued with TV, and over time I did a few things on camera. I'd created a character called 'Peter Puffpaint', which I performed at the Fringe and Midsumma festivals, but I knew this wasn't going to get me anywhere. I decided that—with everything I had been through and the sudden interest we all had in current affairs—being a journalist would be a good career path for me.

I had the sense that the freethinking transcendentalism of the 1990s had flown off somewhere on a unicorn. Little mattered in my life, and the lives of those around me, except career success and finding somewhere nice to live. But it wasn't just that: I now had friends, a relationship, an interest in community radio and TV—in sum, I had a brittle but growing sense of achievement and belonging.

It took me years to get into the media industry. I often wept at how hard it was, how embarrassed I was at having to continue working as a telemarketer at night to support my various low-paying media jobs. With higher ambitions—and without the option of jumping off and falling—my anxiety, and certainly my status anxiety, increased. I felt as if I was two steps behind everyone else; my colleagues were eighteen and nineteen years old, while I was twenty-three and still working part-time in a call centre. I dealt with my anxiety by cutting myself with a knife until my partner told me I needed to get help—so I got a referral to see a psychiatrist in Clayton.

Dr Lennon was a man in his mid-forties with an orange beard and a nice car. Over time, he undoubtedly helped me a lot: I stopped cutting, I got my career on track. He told me that part of improving my life had to involve the delicate balancing act of simultaneously realising that things hadn't gone right in the past, but not sending myself into despair with self-loathing commentary at every step I took. I guess I was looking for a kind of father-figure, with whom I could discuss even practical things—something I had been unable to do with my own dad, whose behaviour had been become increasingly erratic and self-centred after his boss decided to close the abattoir, where he managed the piggery section, just after 2000.

It was fitting, therefore, that Dr Lennon started looking at me—after a while—as if I had just been to the toilet and not washed my hands. Eventually, in his well-crafted accent, he told me that he didn't like the fact I came to therapy without showering, dressing properly, or styling my hair. He cancelled the sessions as soon as I told him I was struggling to pay them, and he immediately sent the remaining debt to a debt collector. I would later get my hands on a progress report he sent to the referring doctor. There was no mention of anything I went through in high school in this letter. Instead, most of it was dedicated to whether or not I had a Borderline Personality Disorder, because while I self-harmed, and had a history of substance abuse (and a 'history of confusion over his sexual identity'), I had shown signs of having both empathy and long-term friendships. In the end, he concluded that I didn't have a BPD.

My partner and I moved into an apartment in the city, and we had a cat, and a nice life by the Yarra. This time would be part of a five-year period during which I didn't take drugs, and so I was unaware, for the most part, that Australia was having its first methamphetamine surge. During this time, Beck moved into a housing-commission house in the country. She got back together with Nick, and gave birth to her second child, another girl, whom she called Alice. Smithy lived all over Melbourne; he had periods of working and then periods of lying on the couch with the curtains closed for a long time. He continued taking 'speed'—as in, powdered meth—on weekends. He was moody, volatile, often charming, and at other times verbally abusive. He met a woman, got her pregnant, and then one day—for reasons he says he does not understand—she snuck away in the middle of the night with their 6-year-old, and never came back.

While all this was happening, I first got a job at the ABC in Ballarat, then Mt Gambier, and then finally as a reporter at triple j. Each of these gave me a confidence boost at the time, but I still didn't feel completely comfortable in my own skin.

My parents, meanwhile, changed a lot during this period. Dad had something of a breakdown after the abattoir closed, and eventually went to the doctor, where he was diagnosed with Bipolar II (the less severe variety). After beginning to take anti-depressants, he found a level of happiness that he hadn't experienced in a long time. Seeing the difference in him, Mum also went to the doctor, and was placed on an anti-depressant that also worked to reduce anxiety. I cannot begin to describe how much Mum changed. She became happy-go-lucky, she grew her hair long, and she was always ringing to see how I was. She was silly, and funny, and was always making jokes. I had never imagined that the reason for her being so aggressive all the time was actually anxiety.

Eventually, my parents moved to Queensland. A few years later, Mum paid for me to go travelling up the east coast of Queensland with her, and I had a marvellous time. Along the way I took her to a few gay clubs, which she in turn experienced as a marvellous time.

I guess things were looking good for us, in some ways. By 2005, I had spent nearly four years without touching a single drug except alcohol.

It was a smarter decision than I realised at the time.

In 2004, experts from both academia and the medical frontline were claiming that the meth problem was at least as large as the heroin peak in the late 1990s. A National Drug and Research Centre (NDARC) study in 2005 suggested there were 73,000 people nationwide addicted to methamphetamine—about 1.5 times the number of heroin addicts. Meth users were also found to have a rate of psychosis 11 times higher than the general population, and many of those had no prior or family history of mental illness.

While crystal meth was then only making up a tiny proportion of meth use, the ACC would warn in its 2004–05 Illicit Drug Data Report that:

> Increasing demand for high purity crystal methylamphetamine, which is readily available in Asia, is likely to create an increase in attempted importation and domestic production in the foreseeable future.

The ACC's 2005–06 Illicit Drug Data Report would follow, stating that: 'Globally, approximately 50 per cent of all global ATS (Amphetamine-type stimulant) production takes place in

East and Southeast Asia, Burma, and China' and that there had been 'a significant increase in the number of ATS laboratories dismantled globally, from 547 in 1990 to 11,253 in 2003'.

Indeed, in winter 2004, long before *Breaking Bad* hit our screens, Fijian police, in collaboration with the Australian and New Zealand authorities, discovered a massive methamphetamine lab hidden in a three-storey building complex near the Fijian capital, Suva. The laboratory had an estimated production capacity of 500 kilograms of crystal methamphetamine a week.

More 'super-labs' would be found in the Philippines, Malaysia, China, and Indonesia over the coming years. Burma would remain the world capital for producing powdered meth pills, also known as Yaba. However, the vast majority of the meth being consumed in Australia was still homemade then, and all of it was powdered meth. Some of it was being made from cold-and-flu tablets obtained from chemists; the rest of it was relying on overseas imports of ephedrine and pseudoephedrine.

Further research from NDARC in 2005 suggested that in some parts of Sydney, the domestic production and supply of meth was entirely controlled by outlaw bikie gangs. But the criminal market was becoming increasingly diversified, fragmented, and difficult to crack — it involved new alliances and new groups. Legitimate businesspeople in Australia were also mixing their lawful activities with forays into the drug trade. Many manufacturers were small-time, and others simply made meth for themselves and a few friends. There was now no set of key groups or individuals that controlled the national meth trade, the links of which often stretched right across Southeast Asia.

So meth — though not yet crystallised meth — was both proving popular and doing damage in the nation. With apologies to Tolstoy — while every meth abuser and addict ends up looking and behaving roughly the same, each has their own reason for getting hooked.

At the beginning of 2007, my life had been steadily improving for five years; I had been drug-free for six. I was clean for a long time. A long time is good, but it is not forever. Despite my good intentions, and despite ticking what I thought were 'life's boxes', at the age of twenty-seven, my life rapidly unravelled. As is characteristic of a breakdown, it seemed like a mess of random events at the time, but looking back now, it all seems patently and painfully logical. This is how it went: I broke up with my partner after a six-year relationship, an amicable and mutual split — we both agreed the relationship had run its course. The apartment felt half empty when he took half the furniture, and entirely empty when he took my beloved cat. I hadn't realised how much of my time and life was taken up by a relationship, and the force of the break-up proved to be bigger than I could handle. I tried going out to clubs, but had little confidence after being in a cozy relationship for so long; I started to feel lost, lonely, and ugly, and felt too intimidated to go out and meet people. When I *did* go out, I started searching for drugs, pills mainly, as soon as I walked in the door. Amphetamines always did the trick; I was able to go up and talk to people without a second thought. The more I looked in the mirror, though, the more I hated what I saw. I had forgotten how often I'd felt like this before I was in a long-term relationship.

It wasn't all bad, though — I also saw the end of the relationship as a chance to have more fun, to date young guys I hadn't had the chance to date when I myself was eighteen and nineteen, and, most importantly, to concentrate on my career. I decided that six years of radio — including two award nominations and getting a job at triple j — would culminate in me getting my own show on Sunday nights over summer. I had been making comedy for triple j's evening show, done some work on its TV show, written for its magazine, and appeared as a guest on nearly every other of its shows. I decided the best way to deal with not having anything to do on weekends was to go to the studio and work on my demo.

The program director called me into his office a month later, saying that he liked the idea for the show, but didn't want me presenting it. I wasn't surprised that he didn't say yes straight away because the demo was, in the end, an over-baked mistake. But his feedback was particularly disheartening: he suggested that I had a 'long, long, long way to go if you want to present a show on the station' but didn't tell me what I needed to improve upon. His attitude seemed to suggest that I was not very good at being a presenter, and that there was very little point in me pursuing this line of career; or, at least, that is how I remember it.

I bought $450 worth of cocaine the weekend after the project failed. In the coming weeks, my feelings of loneliness and rejection morphed into abject feelings of self-disgust. I became so miserable that life felt surreal. I had spent five years building up a radio career, sure that it was my destiny, and now my career—which had been all-important to me—felt like a complete waste of time.

The only relief was drugs, which I had started taking every weekend. At first I took ecstasy, which filled me with hubris, deception, and all things nice. Going to work at my job as a reporter began to seem utterly pointless, and I started taking days off during the week, turning up late, and missing deadlines. Soon, I was going to nightclubs and taking drugs Thursday through Monday every week. By then I was using GHB and ketamine, and when they stopped working, I started smoking meth. I spent all week at work fantasising about being high, which gradually turned into crying at my desk, then having lines at my desk, and then I stopped turning up at work altogether.

For a long while, my weekends were amazing. I went to a now defunct nightclub called The Market—this was just before the emergence of Facebook and smartphones, when people still went out. Thousands packed the place every Friday and Saturday night, from all walks of life, and partied until the place closed at 11.00am on Sunday, amid balloons, streamers, transvestites, and drugs.

I would dance for hours, and talk to strangers all night long. Before things got really bad, I knew that my work performance was seriously dropping, but while I hated getting yelled at, I just didn't care. I had what seems now to be a rather prophetic dream one night that I was on the dance floor at The Market when I realised I had marbles in my pockets, and that I had just spilt them, and that my boss was standing there, hands on hips, demanding I pick them up. I *did* try—but by then they had scattered everywhere.

It was hard for me to imagine, at that point in time, how anybody could get through the week without having a party on the weekend to look forward to; it was certainly the only thing that got me through the week. And as the winter set in, that week took on a slow, sickly rhythm, during which I was tired, and desperate, and obsessing over every second guy I met. There was one who became a full-time obsession; when he didn't text me back, I felt so miserable I would pile on the pills and the meth to forget about him, but when the drugs wore off, he would come back into my mind, bit by bit, until I took more.

The therapists I saw were expensive and didn't seem to get it; I was taking anti-depressants that didn't do much good either. A psychologist I was seeing called a CAT team after I told him that the Zoloft I was prescribed made me feel like stabbing random people at a shopping centre. They told me to see a therapist, to keep taking my anti-depressants, and to stop using drugs.

Work noticed that I was going downhill. They calculated all of the sick leave and annual leave I was owed, and gave me six weeks off. I went to Queensland and stopped using drugs; when I came back, though, I felt depressed also immediately, and starting using again.

When I got back, the ABC sent me to a psychiatrist—as far as I know, it cost them $1,500. But this was not for treatment—which, as I was only working part-time then, I couldn't afford—it was, at HR's initiation, a Fitness for Work Assessment. The report came back with the use of Axis and Criterion (which are the diagnostic tools used by the Diagnostic and Statistical Manual of Mental Disorders (DSM)) to conclude that I had 'Major Depressive Disorder in the context of Substance Abuse and Borderline Personality Traits'.

Meanwhile, I had begun to obsess over guys again: one day, when one of them didn't message me back, I sent him flowers. When he still didn't reply, I took a knife into the work bathroom, and made a long, thin cut from my knee to my groin.

I didn't feel as though I could tell anyone about these humiliations. Whenever I did start to talk to people about what I was going through, I could see them either getting very uncomfortable or they would start lecturing me on what I was doing wrong. That, or they just couldn't have cared less.

At home, I spent hours staring out at the grey Melbourne sky from my high-rise Southbank apartment, miserable and anxious. One day, I decided to give Beck a call; it had been about two years since I had last seen her. As soon as she asked me how I was, it all came pouring out. She listened to everything, and then relayed three or four stories from her own life that seemed to not only encapsulate how I felt, but were remarkably similar to what I had been through. Only Beck, it seemed, had the empathy and the selflessness to admit to having endured the same humiliations as me when it came to unrequited love.

She asked me to come over, and I ended up basically living with her. While there, I met a friend of Nick's—he was by now well and truly off the scene, but his friends still came around—who had recently gotten out of jail. We started a romance as well as starting to use heroin together—never enough to get me addicted, but enough to stop me from killing myself.

I started taking Beck to The Market, where, like everyone else, she had the time of her life. One night, she told me she was going home early because she had bumped into the guy she'd met in a Ferntree Gully pool hall a few weeks earlier, and they were going back to his house to smoke some meth with his two gay mates.

She gave me the key to her place, and returned the next day in a riotous mood. The following weekend, that guy—Rob Smith—was over again, and the weekend after that, and soon enough he hardly left.

From the outset I found 'Smithy', as we called him, to be kind, friendly, down to earth, generous, and very quick to give a compliment. He and Beck hung out together for a good few weeks before they finally slept together, and he seemed—in his own rough way—to be a real gentleman. He came out with just me a few times, and one night we were joined by another friend; we went back to her house and shot up some heroin. I'll never forget him sweating so much that she—on a fairly cold night—took him out to the backyard, and hosed him down with the garden hose. Around the same time, the guy who I had met at Beck's died from a heroin-related illness.

Needless to say, my work was suffering more and more, and I was quickly becoming a liability. Work managers were very supportive until they got the psychiatrist's report—when they realised I was also using drugs, my manager told me I was an 'occupational risk' to other employees (at triple j). I was eventually called into a meeting with HR and my manager, who said if I didn't go to a residential rehab I would almost certainly lose my job; she felt I was underperforming to such an extent that I could be placed under a performance review. She said that over 160 people had applied for my job, and that there were award-winning young journalists who had worked on *7.30* and *Lateline* who had missed out to me—even though I was less qualified—and she was now beginning to believe that she had a mistake. I sobbed loudly in front of them for ten minutes, and agreed that yes, rehab was only the option. I went back to my parents, and in the sunshine and isolation, my need for drugs subsided, and by Christmas of that year I was clean. As a condition of getting my job back, though, I still had to go to residential rehab.

As quickly as methamphetamine use had risen in Australia, it now — almost inexplicably, and without the fanfare of its dramatic introduction — began to drop. According to the 2007 National Drug Strategy Household Survey (NDSHS), the proportion of Australians who reported use of these drugs in the previous twelve months decreased significantly, from 3.2 per cent in 2004 to 2.3 per cent in 2007. The meth scare seemed to be over, and it also seemed as if many people had been guilty of engaging in a bit of moral panic. In fact, ecstasy use was still far higher, and used by far more people, than methamphetamine in 2007. The proportion of Australians who had 'ever used' methamphetamine also decreased significantly, from 9.1 per cent to 6.3 per cent.

Meth's popularity — at least as we understood meth then — seemed to be in free-fall. Perhaps the world had moved on, and the nation's drug users were re-collecting their marbles and going back to work and regular play — including me.

## Chapter Six

# Every creature has its soft spots

IN A CLASS, in a public rehab on the rural outskirts of Brisbane's southern suburbs, Audrey, a thirty-something black New Guinean with a slight, almost European-sounding accent, was telling her group, 'Addiction is an illness, addiction is a coping mechanism. Addiction is about survival.'

Audrey was methodically making eye contact—through her 1960s-style eyeliner—with each of the 11 people in her rehab class. Half were jailbirds who were being forced to attend; there were also two former school teachers, a guy with schizophrenia, a bespectacled middle-aged librarian addicted to sleeping tables, and Richard, the self-described 'bisexual bipolar bear', who was in rehab after neighbours found him trying to gas himself in the car while on amphetamines. Many eyes were drifting off Audrey, onto the gum trees and the farmland out the window, and perhaps to the future (their plans for when they leave), or to the past (the joys and sorrows of drug use).

'The brain associates drugs with pleasure, the opposite of pain and death—but instead of giving yourself something that nourishes you and gives you strength, an addict is engaging in behaviour that will make their life worse in the long run,' Audrey explained. 'You face a problem, you take drugs, your problem gets worse, you take more drugs and on it goes; that is what we call the cycle of addiction.'

Sitting among this motley crew was me: I had arrived three days earlier with my head wrapped in a skull bandana, and my stomach a mess of angry echidnas. I was clean by this stage, and wasn't too keen on going to rehab, or even going back to my job, but the prospect of life on the dole—that is to say, life without parties or drugs while living at my parents' house, an hour away from Bundaberg—didn't grab me either. I *was*, however, keen to work out what had gone wrong, and how I could go back to normal life without experiencing the flood of misery that was my usual experience. I didn't really believe that rehab would help, but I was curious to see if it could.

So in February 2008, Eileen the admin lady picked me up from Beenleigh train station in a minivan. 'It's quite an interesting area around here,' she remarked. 'A few years ago it was all rural; now it's becoming an outer suburb of Brisbane.'

We were actually about half-an-hour's drive from my old haunt of Woodridge, which seemed appropriate. Logan House was a publicly funded rehab; the weekly bill was taken straight out of my Centrelink payments. By way of comparison, the Sanctuary, a luxury private rehab in Byron Bay, costs $30,000 a week, and you can get in straight away. Logan House cost $220 a week. It was a bargain, really; for that we got three meals a day, and about a tenth of the medical staff that are employed by the Sanctuary.

Eileen drove me up the driveway, from where I could see the tennis court and the pool. Like the rest of the buildings, the front office was made of 'he used to give me roses' brown brick.

There were three villas, holding about 24 residents in total, and each of us shared a room with two others.

Eileen explained the rules:

- There was no contact with anybody from the outside for the first twenty-one days.
- Urine and breath tests twice a week.
- The day started at 6.30am with exercise, then classes, four days a week.

Eileen asked if I had deodorant or Listerine or any medications. I answered yes, and she took them off me and put them in a locker, telling me that people can get high on deodorant and Listerine in rehab. I was allowed to keep my asthma medication in my room, but she took my Zoloft from me: I could only take that during specified medication times.

The first resident I met at Logan House was a guy in my villa: he was a talented musician in his early twenties called Max.

'What's your poison?' he said.

'Party drugs; I partied Thursday through Monday,' I replied. 'And eventually heroin on Tuesdays and Wednesdays. Until my managers at my radio job told me to take time off or face the axe.'

'Here sit down, have a smoke with me,' Max said. 'This is how it went wrong for me, dude. My ex-girlfriend and I were supposed to go to Europe together. I started, like, partying and dealing and stuff, and she told me I couldn't come. But that's why I was dealing, so I could save money. Well, she went to Europe and I'm still here, and with all the money I saved, I spent it on heroin.'

A second guy sat down with us, having overheard Max talking. He was tall with brown hair and a deep Scottish accent.

'I had a breakdown,' he said without being prompted. 'And then I went back to the booze.'

'How are you now?'

'Getting there. It's difficult. I've been here six weeks. I've been to rehab before, but I really want to make it this time ... and don't worry, there are lots of educated professionals here, you'll fit right in. There are all kinds of people here: teachers, business owners, musicians, even a psychologist.'

'A psychologist in rehab? You mean as a client?'

'Yep.'

And a few days later I would meet her—her name was Holly—while she was raking up some leaves outside one of the villas. She had brown hair and brown eyes. She told me she became an alcoholic a year or two after her husband died. 'You know, the thing about grief is, the more you hold on to it—the worse it gets,' she said.

Unlike most rehabs, which are based on the 12-step program, the rehab course at Logan was based on cognitive behavioural therapy (CBT); we were taught that our thoughts control our behaviours and emotions, and our willpower controls our thoughts. We would have a weekly one-on-one counselling session, using techniques by which we would learn to expect and tolerate restless or low moods. We learned to question those assumptions that reinforced our habits (for example, 'I'll never make friends who don't do drugs'), and to focus on engaging our non-drug activities and creative interests.

The classes were certainly interesting. We were told that thoughts control everything, and that we had complex psychological reasons for drug triggers. According to Audrey, most of our heartache is caused by our own thinking. She told us that most negative thinking is the result of errors in reasoning; what she called 'thinking distortions', such as 'overgeneralisation', and 'all-or-nothing thinking'.

In class, we discussed triggers and traumas. Men talked about being dumped. A young stripper said she used to get so smashed she would peel her cigarettes and eat them like a banana. We each made a list of events that often led to our drug use. For many people, those triggers were similar: 'Friday nights', 'having an argument with my partner', or 'hearing dance music'. Audrey explained that 'hearing dance music' belongs to a category called 'euphoric recall'. I wrote my list of risky events:

- Being dumped
- Going out
- Being at a venue
- Stressful day at work
- Having something good happen
- Having something bad happen

Audrey was also my individual counsellor. We had our one-on-one sessions by the river once a week. The thing I found most irritating about her was the way she kept about asking about my homosexuality, and whether or not I had been mistreated because of it. At the time, this seemed completely irrelevant to me.

During our first sessions, I told her I was worried that I might seem a bit boring without drugs.

'Boring?'

'Yeah, like when I was a workaholic journalist and a nerd.'

'Luke, if I saw you at a party, I would want to talk to you. You *are* interesting.'

'Are you spinning me a line, Audrey? As in a standard psychology how-to-make-someone-feel-better line?'

'I'm not that sort of counsellor, Luke. From what I've seen of you in class today, I like you a lot. You're a deep thinker, and I think you have a big heart. You have a tough facade to protect yourself, but I think you're very sensitive underneath.'

By our second session, I realised I struggled with group situations, and that my parents had mental-health problems, and so I over-achieved or recklessly under-achieved to get their attention. Audrey asked me to write a list of things I had achieved in life, and to 'take full credit for them'. I have to admit, I started to feel better and more in control of my life after just a few days.

But even still, I was nervous, my thoughts were racing; I couldn't sleep, and all I wanted to do was sleep.

Come week three, and although many people had been listening and agreeing, a dissenter emerged in class. This dissenter was Max, who said, 'Audrey, we keep hearing in class that drugs are the result of a lack of something else in our lives. But lots of people here are confident and seem happy. I just don't think I will ever find the same high I found on drugs anywhere else.'

Although Audrey was quick to disagree, telling Max that that kind of justification was 'cognitive distortion' and that 90 per cent of people with addictions have a mental illness, the damage had been done. I was having a lot of trouble coping without drugs, and Max's line of reasoning made it worse.

I found myself walking around at night: pacing, wanting to leave, hating being there. I couldn't sleep, I was up all night, my mind racing and worrying. I wanted to leave; I felt like an idiot, it felt melodramatic to be there in rehab. I made small incisions with a pair of nail scissors on the inside of my thigh. Halfway through my next counselling session with Audrey, after pushing myself again and again to tell her what I did, I told her that I had cut myself.

She put her hand on my leg. She told me cutting didn't help. I told her I felt that it did. She told me I cut myself when I was anxious, and I needed to do breathing exercises instead. She told me that my thoughts caused my anxiety, and that my thoughts were things I could control. She told me there was no need for me to be anxious. She said I was funny, and attractive, and smart. She told me I was safe.

'Anxiety comes in waves,' she said. 'It peaks and then it goes. You need to identify when it is starting, and slow down your breathing. When you slow down your breathing, your body will relax, and you will feel better. You don't need to cut yourself to feel better.'

Audrey then took me into the director's office. Apparently, an episode of self-harm was considered a serious incident in rehab. The director was a tall, strong-looking woman with greying hair cut in a kind of flat-top.

'Luke, self-harm is a maladaptive way of dealing with anxiety,' she said. 'Your body is preparing itself to fight or to run when it senses danger. You are becoming aggressive when you feel anxious, but you are turning your aggression on yourself. It's not actually helping your situation to cut yourself. Do you understand what I mean?'

'I think so,' I replied.

'You feel scared or worried about something, you can't cope, so you lash out at yourself,' she said.

And suddenly I *did* understand; the concept of internalised aggression made perfect sense. It was what we called in rehab a 'light-bulb moment', and the urge to self-harm started to dissipate thereafter.

But I still felt anxious, and I still had trouble sleeping. Audrey asked again and again whether I was comfortable with my sexuality, and I began to resent her for it.

More classes followed. We talked about boundaries, and the ways in which they can be violated: physically, sexually, socially, emotionally, psychologically, and spiritually.

The vast majority of people relapse shortly after they leave rehab, whether they finish the program or not. Many people fail at rehab. One patient asked nearly everybody—including me and including all the staff—for sex. It was near constant, and he was eventually kicked out. The librarian was expelled a short time later for smuggling in anti-psychotics, and taking them in the morning, so she could sleep all day and avoid class. A few weeks later, a resident with schizophrenia left in the middle of the night, bought some heroin, found a syringe, injected it and died almost instantly—a reasonably common problem among addicts when they leave rehab, and, after having had a break from their drug, take a dose that is far too high for what their body is now used to.

But there are also people who graduate and stay clean. Holly, the psychologist, graduated the eight-week program. Her mother and daughter attended the graduation, beaming with smiles. Before she left, she thanked the girls in her villa for 'making me feel beautiful again'.

And me? Well, I still couldn't sleep. And I was still annoyed at why Audrey kept asking me whether or not I was comfortable with my sexuality. One night, my annoyance with her turned into an extensive diary entry about high school—the first time I had written any of it down. When I had my next session with Audrey, she became the first person I told what had happened at high school.

She gently rubbed my back as I went through all the details; I sobbed, but by the time I'd finished, I had become angry.

'You've got through the worst of it,' Audrey told me. 'You have already survived it; it's time now to accept yourself and be kinder to yourself.'

I stayed awake all the next night, feeling tender and exposed; a soft spot had been uncovered.

I learnt a lot about soft spots during my time in rehab. That started when I saw a guy named Billy punching a boxing bag. He looked like Rocky; he had a boxer's nose, and was Italian or Greek, and he was really going at it. I knew he had just spent a fair bit of time in jail, but he was actually pretty friendly, and when he saw me walking past he called me over.

He said he used to be a competitive boxer, and asked if I had ever boxed before. I laughed nervously and said no. He got a pair of boxing gloves for me, and proceeded to show me the basics of how to throw a punch.

'Turn your arm as you do it, so it's all knuckle,' he said. Self-consciously, I started hitting the bag again and again until I found a rhythm, and I ended up doing it for about half an hour.

We had a few more boxing sessions after that. And then, the day after my big day with Audrey, Max came up to me, announcing he had come up with a plan for me, inspired by a highly effeminate champion Thai kickboxer he once saw on TV.

'I am going to turn you into society's worst nightmare,' he said.

'What's that?'

'A poof who can kill.'

'No, Max,' I said. 'I don't need to know that kind of thing, not anymore.'

'C'mon,' he protested. 'It will give you confidence.'

So he took me into the shed with the boxing bag.

His philosophy was simple — your hard bits thrown at full force to the other person's soft bits.

Elbows to eye sockets.

Knees to testicles.

Fists to windpipe.

Shin to stomach.

Legs to ribs.

Head to back of head.

And so on.

Even with all this activity, I couldn't sleep, so the rehab took me to the doctor. I was prescribed anti-psychotics, and woke up after weeks of not sleeping properly, light as a feather with a peace I had never known before: fear could be overcome, failure was simply a matter of perception, demons had been slayed, and there was a light shining out of my heart.

I wrote this note in my diary:

I go back to my room. I think about, for some strange reason, Easter, and I thought about boundaries. What is in my boundary? I thought. Me, self-love, me, good stuff, me, me, me. I start feeling a strange sensation in my chest. Perhaps it's some epithet of narcissism, but it feels like something else. It feels like I've tapped into some kind of divine energy. I feel a little white light or something glowing out of me. I feel connected with all the living things around me. I think about Jesus Christ. I never got the myth of Jesus, it never made any sense. Now it seems to have kind of clicked. It's like no matter what suffering and hatred we endure in life, we will always rise up because we will always have our essence. We can all rise again cos nothing ever kills our essence.

I am not saying I want to be a Christian, no way, but I understand the spiritual messages of Christianity now. But it feels right. And it feels like for the first time, maybe I have grasped what it means to have a soul.

I woke that day feeling light and lovely, feeling as if anything at all—including complete sobriety—was now within my reach.

Then suddenly my time was up. I gave a goodbye talk to the group, in which I revealed I had cried over things that happened to me fifteen years ago. I told them I'd recognised that my drug abuse was a form of poorly expressed, internalised rage. Everyone clapped, and I left. It felt life-changing, revelatory; nothing could stop me, anything could be achieved.

Meanwhile, methamphetamine use had continued on its downward fall, which began toward the end of 2005 and went on right until 2011.

In 2010, at 2.1 per cent across the population, use of methamphetamines had fallen to the lowest level seen since 1995. A similar trend was seen among young people, where students were less likely to have ever used the drug in 2011 (2.9 per cent) than in 2005 (5.3 per cent). Clandestine-lab detections had also dropped, as had meth imports and drug offences.

There was a sense—at least in drug circles, and by following what the media were saying—that meth had come and gone. However, others—and by others I mean here experts in the field—were less convinced. They tended to see the drop-off in meth use as either 1) too insignificant to be statistically meaningful or 2) simply part of what many see as the inherently cyclical nature of population drug epidemics.

'Drugs, for a number of different reasons, come in and out of fashion all the time,' Geoff Munro, national policy manager with the Australian Drug and Alcohol Foundation, told me. 'There will always be a population cohort of addicts who abuse the strongest drug they can find; drugs throughout history follow an often inexplicable cycle of being widely abused, and then use falls off again, before we get another spike a few years or a decade later.'

According to the cyclical perspective on community drug 'epidemics', the dynamic nature of drug markets—both supply and demand—means that today's problem drug could well be replaced by a new problem drug tomorrow.

Another possible reason for the decrease in use was the tightening of restrictions governing the sale of pseudoephedrine-based cold-and-flu tablets in some states. Most meth being consumed in Australia in that decade (2000–10) was being made here, and intelligence suggested most manufacturers were sourcing their precursor material through 'pseudoephedrine runners' who went from chemist to chemist all over the state, and sometimes interstate, to buy cold-and-flu tablets in bulk. Queensland, perhaps because of its vast geography and scattered populations, has always been Australia's meth-making capital. So in November 2005, the Queensland state government brought in Project Stop, an electronic tool and database that allowed for sales of pseudoephedrine to be tracked in real time using a Global Positioning System. This system aimed to prevent individuals from purchasing small quantities of pseudoephedrine from many different pharmacies. In the short term, the project seemed to work; the number of clandestine labs in Queensland dropped between 2005 and 2007 by 23 per cent. By 2006, nationally, all products containing pseudoephedrine had been rescheduled as either 'Pharmacist Only Medicines' (Schedule 3) or 'Prescription Only Medicines' (Schedule 4), depending on the amount of pseudoephedrine in the product. This means that prior to 2005, anybody could buy pseudoephedrine off the shelves without asking a pharmacist, or showing ID, let alone getting a prescription. Given that nearly all meth is made with either ephedrine or pseudoephedrine, it's not surprising that many people were taking advantage of this loophole. Jason Ferris, a senior research fellow at the University of Queensland, has extensively studied Project Stop, and told me that a national compulsory system would reduce the opportunities for addict-based manufacturers to make meth.

However, others, such as the ACC, have suggested that the tighter controls on pseudoephedrine simply resulted in the growth of the illicit-precursor importation market. Indeed, the US introduced the federal Combat Methamphetamine Epidemic Act in 2005, which increased restrictions on pseudoephedrine sales. Similarly to Australia, pharmacists and sellers of medications containing pseudoephedrine were required to place these medications behind the counter, and buyers were required to show a state-issued identification card and sign a log that could be used to track their purchases. Two researchers, Dobkin and Nicosia, studied the effect of this legislation, and concluded that this intervention substantially disrupted the supply of methamphetamine, but that the effect was only temporary.

All things considered, this legislation may have opened up a market for more sophisticated meth manufacturers overseas and here. Meth's minor drop-off at the end of last decade turned out to be the calm before the storm—from where we are now, we can see that Australia's meth story goes something like this: The first clouds of meth were detected in the syringes of Sydney's injecting drug users in the mid-1990s. Then came the thunder—crime bosses across Asia stopped producing heroin, and started making the profitable, easier-to-make methamphetamine in 1999. Local drug dealers and crime gangs got on board and starting making gear; as a result, it rained powdered meth in Australia from mid-2000 to mid-2004. Then things dried up. Years later, without any apparent warning and before we had a chance to notice the dark clouds, it started raining crystal hail.

And before the storm, and after rehab, I was back living at Beck's.

Rehab is a bit like an idealised society, where you don't have the usual life and money pressures. When I returned to real life, I was relegated to part-time work because of my breakdown; I couldn't afford my own place, and my family lived in Queensland, and couldn't help me. So I wasn't really able to cut ties with the only people who could offer me a cheap room: people who were always using drugs. That is to say, Beck—and Beck's place was now hers *and* Smithy's.

I returned to work in Melbourne. While I never reached the same levels of misery and low self-esteem, and my life was without a doubt better after I got out of rehab, I still fell back into addiction. Non-drug-using people tended to avoid me, and I them; I continued hanging out with my drug-using friends instead. We smoked pot most nights, and some mornings, and on Friday nights, we snorted powdered meth.

And these Friday nights were undoubtedly the best night of the week because everyone was so happy and upbeat. But the meth was so weak then—this was back in 2008–09—that I found it easy not to use; when I *did* use, I usually fell asleep, and when I woke up the next day I always regretted it because I had less energy in the gym—though I still went. I didn't really go out, because living with Beck and Smithy meant that I felt less lonely.

Smithy and Beck, meanwhile, had settled into a life together: a life of silly jokes, bad TV, and drugs. During the week, Beck would yell and scream. Smithy would take at least one day a week off work—usually on Tuesday or Wednesday—when he would literally just lie there awake, staring at the wall, and wouldn't answer if you spoke to him. He dealt bits and bobs of pot to make ends meet.

Smithy *did* bring an element of stability to the household, if for no other reason than that he actually did work (apart from those mid-week days off). He also loved sport, and went to work quickly to ensure both of Beck's daughters played sport. He went along and watched their games every week, and referred to both of them as 'champions'.

With a more stable household, Beck always offered a couch to anybody who needed it (and in my case a room to someone who needed it). One day a woman from the neighbourhood said she was going through some issues and dropped off her cat. Beck took George—a cat with a gimpy leg—in, no questions asked.

Later, the same would happen with somebody's dog. The dog had a large cyst on its face, and Beck sat by the heater with the dog, squeezed the entire cyst out onto a tissue, and cleaned it up with antiseptic—the cyst never grew back. A short time later, somebody dropped off *another* dog, which got the first dog pregnant. The male dog was then adopted out, and the female died during birth. Beck bottle-fed the puppies for the first six weeks, setting her alarm every six hours. She gave away three of the puppies, and kept one for herself—that dog is now seven, and as far as I know, it still lives with Smithy.

But all was not well in Beck's world, and by the time she reached the age of thirty, it was beginning to show. I'm not sure exactly when it started, but she began to experience a smouldering resentment towards others and the world, which, over time, became an obsessive, perhaps pathological, jealousy.

Beck regarded anybody who had any measure of success with open disdain, and sometimes subjected them to abuse—and she had an extremely wide definition of success. She regarded my achievements as a mere consequence of my parents having money, or the fact that I received private tuition, or the two years I had spent at a private school.

It wasn't just people from our general area who had gone on to have money (or mediocre journalism careers) that Beck resented; it was anybody who had a mortgage or a nice car. One day, in Coles, she commented that the 'women working in the deli are up themselves' and the gay guy who supervised the checkout area was also 'stuck-up'.

The only jobs she worked as an adult were as a factory-hand, or on a production line in the slowly disappearing manufacturing industry of a rapidly changing Dandenong. When I asked her why she hated all the people who worked in the supermarket, she explained that she had applied for a traineeship a few years back at Coles, and after a day-long workshop-style selection process, she was rejected because she had 'poor group skills', didn't listen and 'constantly talked over the top of people'.

'Too socially retarded to even be a check-out chick,' she said one day, giggling, when she was stoned.

Beck was still funny—even delightful—when she was stoned, and was super-friendly and happy on those Friday nights. In between, though, life could be pretty grim—especially for her kids. Beck's sense of unfairness about how her life had panned out was, after a while, being taken out on her children every morning, as if she had been unfairly sentenced to living in a small house with a partner who slept in a separate room, and two children who she often couldn't stand. Beck's weekday mornings were unpleasant for her, and even more unpleasant for her children after two years of using powdered meth every weekend. The problem was yelling and screaming, and a mood that seemed to have no discernible cause but manifested itself in huffiness and screams of 'fucking hurry up you little cow', 'move it', 'who drank all the milk, there's no fucking milk' before refusing to take her daughters to school, and making Smithy crawl out of bed to drive them. Beck went from waking up with no energy to smashing dishes with such panic-driven hysteria that her youngest would often go to school in anguished tears.

I am not sure why I never said anything; I often heard it, and I was usually glad it wasn't directed at me. I guess we all just sort of got used to it, and tried to stay out of her way.

By about midday, when the kids were at school and Beck had had some more sleep, and smoked some marijuana, she was marvellous again. Witty, funny, offering to get Smithy and me something from the bakery. Whatever we asked for, she would come back with twice as much. I believed that Beck wouldn't have behaved like that if she was fully in control of herself, and I understood why she had a degree of anger—whether in good or bad faith—about the way things had panned out for her in life. If I gently raised the issue of her anger, most of the time she would claim she was 'crook' because she had a cold.

Roughly every second Saturday, Smithy would go out with some mates, and Beck would call him and call him. He'd say he would be fifteen minutes, and would then be away for six hours—with her car. It was as if he liked being out with a man-friend, and having her call every ten minutes, and not answering her calls. That way he could tell his mate—or perhaps just leave the impression—'bitch wants me'. It was unclear to me, though, whether she wanted her car, him, the drugs he said he was buying, or all three.

Amid all this, Beck got pregnant for the third time in just over two years; Smithy was convinced she was deliberately getting herself pregnant to 1) keep him at home more (she used to call him dozens of times and cry for hours on end if he was out for too long on the weekend) and 2), and more importantly in his eyes, to get a financial claim on his father's estate, which by now was worth several million dollars. Smithy was incredulous when Beck got pregnant the third time and urged her to have another abortion. 'Urged' might actually be too nice a way of putting it: Smithy told Beck that if she *didn't* have an abortion this time, he would leave. She cried for days on end, before agreeing that she would give herself a miscarriage by injecting herself with an enormous dose of powdered meth. When she went to the doctor a short time later, she found that not only was her attempt unsuccessful, but also that she was having twin boys. She sat me down in the lounge room when she got home and said, 'I want to have these kids because being a parent is the only thing I am good at.' She promised Smithy that he could be the stay-at-home parent, and she would go and work fulltime at her job packing boxes at a factory. He agreed, and eventually he seemed quite taken with the idea of twin boys. Excited, even—but he made no plans to give up his party lifestyle.

In September 2009, two splendid little beings were born, and brought with them hope, and sunshine, and giggles, and all things that babies give, no matter who their parents are, and no matter what the circumstances of their birth.

Meanwhile, my work situation had become untenable. One day, I got a call from a friend who worked on the same program as me, doing the same job, but who had started about two years later. A top guy, he'd called to ask me why I hadn't applied to present any programs over the summer because, he thought, I would be a very good presenter. He said management needed people to present shows, and when he'd asked to present, he'd been given a heap of graveyard shifts, and—here is the clincher—he didn't need to put in a demo. The next day, I emailed the program director to ask if he needed anybody to do shifts over summer, and whether he needed a demo. He said no, he didn't need anybody, and upon that I got up, walked out of the ABC, and never went back. I took multiple legal actions, won some, lost some, and won enough to get me a big trip to Europe, where, inspired by the fact my legal actions had been more successful than my radio career, I took up a law degree.

By this stage, I was fuming—I felt as if my life had been derailed over and over again by people who had abused their power and screwed me over for no good reason. I was convinced that the reason this has happened was simply because I hadn't been powerful enough. I read my law studies like a madman, and enrolled in boxing (which by then had replaced self-harming as an outlet for anger—but like most things I became obsessed with it and at times I took it too far). I began using steroid cream, and packed on a heap of muscle, which led to heavy weight-lifting and Muay Thai kickboxing, eventually training with competitive teams.

I became very volatile and vicious—looking back, I was not a very nice person a lot of the time. I not only didn't take shit from anybody, but the slightest provocation would see me with my hands around someone's neck, and/or an email to them explaining that I had initiated legal action. By the time I got halfway through my legal studies, several people I knew had employed me as their pro-bono legal advocate (not as a lawyer) in workplace injury, bad loans, and unfair dismissal. They did this knowing I would charge into conciliations and trials using a combination of broadcasting skills, legal know-how, bitchiness, vengeance, and testosterone to scare their adversaries into handing over money.

I was eventually so angry that I would, on occasion, be walking down the street and start punching the Christ out of a tree. In the end, I had to wind things back, as being in a constant state of rage aggravated a neck injury that I had gotten at the ABC; I had to take long periods off from studying law because I was in pain and depressed. I still smoked pot and did a bit of powdered meth, but only to help me focus and prepare for the next battle.

For the most part, Smithy and Beck—along with my parents—were the only people I didn't fight with. By midway through 2011, in fact, Smithy had been spending more and more time on those Friday nights chatting with me while Beck was in bed (she always crashed early). We talked about all manner of things, mainly sport, and he was almost certainly my closest friend for a long while. Over time, however, something curious happened. He stopped talking about sport and started talking about sex.

In particular, he asked me over and over again what I thought about when I masturbated. Usually I would just pretend to go to sleep, and not answer him, but he persisted for months and months. It seemed really grubby and childish to me.

The final straw came late in 2011, the day my alarm went off on the opposite side of the house to Smithy, and he started bitching and mumbling. I had had enough. I walked into his room and told him, in great detail, what I thought of him: he was a fat, lazy, sleazy piece of shit who had done nothing with his life. At the end of the tirade, as he sat there stunned, I gave him a decent shove. Then *he* got mad.

He grabbed me and effortlessly—the guy hadn't done any exercise or work in two years, but was still as strong as an ox—threw me to the ground. He got on top of me, and held both my arms to the ground as I struggled to get up, tearing a muscle in my shoulder in the process. Beck walked in, saw the scene, and screamed, 'I am sick of you coming here, causing trouble between me and Smithy; get out!' So I did, and I didn't speak to either of them for two years after that.

I moved to St Kilda; I found anti-depressants that actually worked; I calmed down, and my neck pain went away. I saw three therapists in this time; the first told me that my rage came from a narcissist's sense of entitlement because of my 'narcissistic personality traits'; the second told me that I nearly met the criteria for an anti-social personality disorder; and finally I found a softly spoken African-American who sent me inside the dreams I had in which I was falling off something. Through this process, I realised that the object I was falling from was life itself, and that when the going got tough, I decided to jump off.

This period when I was away from Smithy and Beck, doing my own thing, was a largely positive one for me. Between 2011 and 2013 — although I still had the odd marijuana and MDMA binge — I finished my law degree, got a job in a community legal centre as a media officer, and was nominated for a Human Rights Media Award for my long-form written journalism. The more I wrote, the better I felt. I started getting paid good money for my print journalism. And, gradually, my dreams changed, too; now when I dreamt I was falling off something, I grew wings. At least once a week I would have a lucid dream in which I flew all over the country, and then deep into the galaxy: when I wrote, I felt as if I could fly.

This feeling of flying was becoming more common, for different reasons, around Australia.

From around 2011 onwards, we had what was basically a new drug on the market — crystallised meth, which was far stronger and far more addictive than the powdered meth that most of us knew only as speed. So it's not surprising that by the reporting period of 2012–13, every state and territory reported an increase in the median purity of methamphetamine. Victoria reported the highest annual median purity of 76.1 per cent in this reporting period, the highest median purity reported in the previous decade—a massive jump when you consider that in 2007 it had dipped to around 17 per cent in most states across the nation. As criminal networks and drug manufacturers got smarter, though, even the powdered meth on the market was of an exceptionally high purity.

On one level, the explanation is simple—more of the drug was getting into the country, and that's because more of it was being made all around the world from around 2011 onward. The cause of our current crystal-meth problem is that so much of the drug is coming through our border, while local production has also risen—as indicated through the detection of clandestine labs—but at a much smaller rate. A few years ago, it was thought that 90 per cent of the meth being used here was locally made; today, that figure is thought to be around 60 per cent.

As Australians grew tired of powdered meth by the mid-2000s, our local dealers seem to have fallen 'victim' to the forces of globalisation—a higher-quality imported product, produced at a cheaper cost. Crystallised meth is now being made all over the world: in the jungles of Burma, in the densely populated slums of Manila, in the deserts of Nigeria, and, perhaps most importantly, in the shantytowns of China. Australia was seen as an easy market for these producers, and soon our hospital emergency rooms were awash with wide-eyed, psychotic meth users.

How exactly did this happen? We need to back up a few steps, and examine what took place in the sub-regions of East and South-East Asia in the first decade of the millennium. For an overview, we can start with these four points, taken from the United Nations Office on Drugs and Crime (UNODC) World Drug Reports from 2008 to 2010:

- While opium cultivation levels worldwide had also restored to and stabilised at pre-2000 levels, drug manufacturers and users were showing a preference for synthetic stimulants. Global seizures of amphetamines increased some threefold over the period 1998–2010, far more than the increases for plant-based drugs.

- In 2008, UNODC reported that methamphetamine use and production was starting to rise, and that 55 per cent of the world's 14 million amphetamine users were in Asia, most of those in the East and Southeast sub-region.
- In the same year, more and more industrial-scale meth labs were being discovered across South-East Asia, 'run by large criminal organisations' according to the UN. By 2009, China accounted for the majority of reported methamphetamine laboratories seized in East and South-East Asia.
- The 2009 UNODC report concluded that Amphetamine-type stimulant (ATS) producers adapt to evade law enforcement. There are signs that criminal organisations are adapting their manufacturing operations to avoid control by: 1) utilising precursor chemicals not under international control; 2) moving manufacturing operations to more vulnerable locations; and 3) shifting precursor chemicals and drug trafficking routes to new locations to avoid detection.

By 2010, there were an increasing number of countries reporting methamphetamine seizures—by now, West African nations were well and truly on board as places to manufacture and distribute drugs, as well as to launder drug money. Iran, Syria, and Pakistan—all of which already had big markets for the legitimate use of crystal-meth precursor drugs—were also developing large black markets. Although the proportion of people requiring treatment for amphetamine abuse was just 5 per cent in Africa, 10 per cent in Europe, and 12 per cent in the Americas, UNODC would report that the number of people seeking treatment was 'particularly high in Oceania (20 per cent) and Asia (21 per cent), reaching 36 per cent in East and South-East Asia with proportions exceeding 50 per cent in Japan, the Republic of Korea, Thailand, Cambodia and the Philippines, as well as in Saudi Arabia in the Near and Middle East' and that 'Government experts have reported that methamphetamine ranks among the top three illicit drugs consumed in several countries in this region, including China, Japan, and Indonesia'.

Although the proportion of people treated for crystal-meth use in Indonesia was far lower, at around 25 per cent, this still signified an increase of almost 80 per cent from the previous year. Crystal-meth users also accounted for the second-largest share of newly admitted patients receiving drug treatment in 2013 at 31 per cent, after heroin users who accounted for a 36 per cent share. Moreover, in China, crystal-meth users accounted for 70 per cent of synthetic drug users receiving treatment in 2013, while methamphetamine tablet users accounted for about 16 per cent.

And it was Asian nations that would continue to drive production, distribution, and demand: and further, it was the growth of richer, younger, more urbanised populations in these nations that was a driving force behind the increase of meth use. These were societies where new opportunities were growing exponentially, and there was a perception that hard work — and having the ability to put in very long days with little sleep — would pay off.

'It originated as a drug that was taken by poor people, traditionally workers. That migrated into youth culture over a decade ago,' Jeremy Douglas, UNODC regional representative for South-East Asia and the Pacific, said in a press statement in 2014. 'More recently, that has evolved into a growing prosperous youth culture … You have rising incomes occurring across the region. You have a large, large youth population. So you have natural growth of the market.'

As these, particularly South-East Asian, nations became richer, and their populations skewed younger, consumer demand for strong amphetamines increased. Between 2008 and 2013, crystal-meth seizures in the entire Asian region almost doubled, while methamphetamine tablet seizures rose at an even more rapid rate, resulting in a seven-fold increase. In November 2013, an ACC report, 'Patterns and Trends of Amphetamine-Type Stimulants (ATS) and Other Drugs—Challenges for Asia and the Pacific 2013', said that:

> Seizures of methamphetamine in both pill and crystalline forms reached record highs [in Asia] in 2012, with 227 million methamphetamine pills seized—a 60 per cent increase from 2011 and a more-than seven-fold increase since 2008—along with 11.6 metric tonnes of crystalline methamphetamine, a 12 per cent rise from 2011.

In its submission to the 2015 Australian federal parliamentary inquiry, UNODC would write that the 'rapidly developing chemical and pharmaceutical industries' in Asia posed a serious threat:

> There is evidence of domestic production in most of the countries of the region, but two countries have advantages that allow them to undercut local prices. The first is Myanmar, where political instability in Shan State and the Special Regions adjoining China has provided cover for large-scale drug manufacturing and trafficking. The second is China, where large quantities of precursor chemicals are produced domestically and industry scale of methamphetamine labs have been continuously dismantled. Myanmar, however, does not have a legitimate pharmaceutical industry, which means

practically that precursor chemicals such as ephedrine and pseudoephedrine must be smuggled from outside Myanmar for the production of methamphetamine. Therefore, precursors have been smuggled from neighbouring countries with large pharmaceutical industries including India and China, whereas the finished methamphetamine products have been trafficked in the reverse direction.

Dr Alex Wodak, from the Australian Drug Law Reform Foundation, told me that drug manufacturing reflected not just an increasingly globalised and outsourced international capitalist economy, but also an economy that creates vast inequality in developing nations, with slick skyscrapers and shopping centres growing around slums, stalls, and beggars.

'People are joining the drug trade to get a slice of this pie,' he said.

In a 2015 report, among the 95 countries and territories worldwide identified as destinations for the meth ATS seized between 2009 and 2013, three of the five most frequently mentioned ones were located in East and South-East Asia and Oceania: Australia, Japan, and Malaysia.

The ACC's CEO Chris Dawson explained to me that the way the world markets for methamphetamine and crystal methamphetamine work are similar to traditional markets—that is, they function according to supply and demand. The supply has increased significantly in recent years because there are more transnational organised crime groups in the market.

Crime groups with international links to the Middle East and Asia have also demonstrated the ability to manufacture and traffic methylamphetamine and its precursor chemicals into Australia. Australia has for several decades had a relatively high level of demand for illicit stimulants, and illicit-drug users in this country pay a premium for illicit drugs compared to their overseas counterparts. This has made Australia an attractive market for transnational crime groups.

And somewhere along the line, probably around the southern summer of 2011–12, Beck and Smithy stopped taking powdered meth, and started taking crystal meth.

Come 2013, and Beck rang me to say she was well and truly over our fight, and she missed me. By now I felt exactly the same, and I told her that. She started visiting me again in my new pad in St Kilda. She told me she had moved into a nice new four-bedroom house in the Toomuc Valley—'new Pakenham … I've finally made it in life'—and that Smithy was also over it. He knew I wasn't very well at the time, and was busting for me to come down. But I stayed away, for whatever reason. While I *did* want to be friends with Smithy again, it just felt too awkward.

Not long after we started talking again, Beck rang me to say she was so sick of Smithy's weird, sleazy games, and his whinging, and his verbal abuse that she had tried to hit him with a toaster. He had gotten a restraining order against her. She moved into another house in the Toomuc Valley, on the cusp of the 100-metre stay-away mark, and, bit by bit, the two started spending time together again.

## Chapter Seven

# Ridgey didge

A FLOCK OF white cockatoos screeched as they flew across the horizon; it seemed as if they had fallen from the last white clouds that remained in the sky's west. The sun was beginning to set, and the clouds surrounding it looked as if a toddler had spilled pink, yellow, and purple paint all over a perfectly blue canvas, which now threatened to drip to the ground. It would only be a few more moments before the night would wipe the sky clean. It was the autumn of 2014, and it was dusk in the Toomuc Valley. Deep in one of the suburb's terracotta-coloured houses, the blind was shut, the lights were off, but Beck was there in her lounge room—just around the corner from Smithy's—staring at the television. Crystal meth had well and truly taken hold of certain sub-sections within the community, Beck among them.

Gravity—or perhaps more specifically, *reality*—had been treating Beck rather harshly all day. In fact, Beck had only fallen from paradise—the crystal-meth high—a few hours earlier, and now the forbidden fruit which had gotten her there was rotting at her heart; she was tumbling, weakened, in freefall. In her own mind, she was a passive victim of this imminent crash—perhaps she was getting sick, perhaps something had infected her.

There was a sensation digging like a butter knife at the base of her skull, and the more she concentrated on it, the more it felt like two sharp screws in her temples, and now she noticed it was blurring her vision as if she were slightly drunk.

Not helping matters was the odour of cat shit coming from the other end of the house. It hit her nostrils only occasionally, and yet it was, to her, a definitive smell: the smell of waste, the smell of something which been kept inside all day. Beck was worried that she would need to put her poor old cat down soon—it had been going to the toilet inside almost every day. Probably, she'd concluded, because the old boy was starting to go senile.

She wished she could be bothered getting up to get her phone. Smithy might have been getting more gear tonight. Meth—make that crystal meth—would have been a spectacularly useful 'pick me up', especially as she thought she was coming down with a flu, and the kids had made a mess of the house, and the stray cat she took in ten years ago was now shitting everywhere, and 'I have to fucking cook dinner tonight', and Smithy had probably given her less than he was supposed to the night before—like he always did, even though she put out, and did 'all the dirty, disgusting things' he wanted her to—and, in fact, Smithy had probably given her share to Luke when she wasn't looking, that was why Luke 'bloody well moved in there in the first place'.

And right at that moment, there was a knock at the door. It was Luke; in other words—me.

I had walked over from Smithy's—a walk which took no more than a few minutes—with something on my mind: a life-changing revelation that had been baking inside my head all day during my own slow drift down from a high. One particular idea was stuck in my head; I felt like a child who'd gotten on a Gravitron before realising I was going to get more than I'd bargained for. When I walked into Beck's house, the first thing I noticed was the aforementioned smell, and just as I came into the room, Beck picked up her iPad and started playing her favourite game—*Zombie Apocalypse*. Her forehead was deeply creased, like a plant that had not been watered for a long time; she had bags under her eyes, and lines on top of those bags. She also had a rather ominous-looking open sore, which had taken up one corner of her chin, and ran roughly half the length of her lips. It was weeping pus, and bleeding slightly. Her shoulders were slumped over. Her eyes seemed darker than normal, and bloodshot; they reminded me of a syringe when its water is mixed with blood.

'Beck, mate, there is something I have to tell you.'

'Mmmm?'

'It's about Smithy,' and at the mention of his name, her face lit up a little. 'I've been in a real panic; I think Smithy has been fucking me, y'know. He hasn't really been giving me meth; he's been giving me acid, and everyone has been laughing at me behind my back. He just took $700 off me; he knew I would say yes because I was on acid. Because I have been getting in all these vortexes, y'know, and wanking constantly, and I've never had meth which has done this before and I think it's because he's charging me for meth and just giving me acid trips and I think everyone is in on it.'

And on I went—and on and on—and Beck's expression didn't change much, but her ears pricked up each time I mentioned Smithy. Eventually, she interjected with, 'Smithy is a psychopath, Luke, he would have done that.'

'Has he, Beck?'

'I don't know, maybe. Stealing money is the kind of thing he would do. Ring him, Luke. Ring him and tell him what you think is going on.'

And so she handed me the phone, having already dialled the number, and said, 'Ask him, ask him.'

'Hello,' Smithy answered in his deep, gravelly voice.

'Smithy, I gave you $100 last night,' I said. 'And I didn't feel shit; it's nothing like the meth I had the other week, I feel like shit now.'

'I fucking told you it was shit gear, you gave me the money anyway,' he said.

'Here's my theory, Smithy—you took my portion, and then gave me acid instead,' and then I left a long silence, waiting for him to put his foot in it.

Emboldened, I took a deeper jab. 'Go on Smithy, I'm listening,' I said.

'How could you fucking say that about me, you are supposed to be my friend, fuck you, you are a fucking arsehole. I gave you acid the other day, remember, does it feel like this meth does?'

And I think honestly and deeply, and I guess it doesn't …

'Well, does it?' he asked.

'No,' I said, realising that this was yet another paranoid delusion that had built up, bit by bit, over the day.

'And you didn't give me $100, you gave me $700—and that was for rent and drugs in advance—remember?'

'Oh,' I said, as my panic turned to relief and then to guilt. 'I'm sorry, seems I got a bit paranoid. Can we perhaps just put this one behind us?'

Smithy started laughing and said, 'I'll see you later on, we need to go and get more gear.'

My fear having been alleviated, all I could sense was the smell of shit, as Beck explained that her cat had gone senile. The odour was becoming unbearable; I got up and followed the smell to find a sloppy, mousse-like turd on the floor of the bathroom. There were a few blowflies buzzing around it. The cat ran up to me—poor old George, the ginger cat with the gimpy foot that Beck had taken in—and started meowing around my legs. I noticed all the doors were shut, so I opened one, and he immediately ran outside and started pissing like a hose. *George wasn't senile at all*, I thought. Beck hadn't been opening the door for him. More to the point, she didn't need to get him put down. Beck—in her state—was undoing all her good deeds.

I cleaned up after the cat, and went back into the lounge room, where I sat on the couch next to Beck. Tears fell down my cheeks. Beck saw this, and turned back to her iPad.

'People were just so horrible to me, for no reason, no fucking reason. I had so many friends, Beck, everyone liked me—and then suddenly nobody would be my friend—nobody!' I said.

My sobbing turned into howling, and upon hearing this, Beck put down her iPad and picked up her book—a second-hand geology book about the structure and metamorphosis of rocks. Something seemed to have drained out of Beck; it seemed to have drained out of the ever-growing hole in her arm. She was so sick of giving a fuck. Nobody ever gave a fuck about her. Nobody ever stuck up for her, patted her on the back when she talked about the torment she had experienced. The same people who picked on her went on to have careers, mortgages, husbands, and twice as many Facebook friends.

She believed that all my paranoia was a symptom of my narcissism; that I wanted everything to revolve around me. Her facial expression had moved slowly over the hour from fatigued to embittered. She was still reading her book on rocks, which was now half covering her face. I had a feeling of clarity, as if I had been working on a maths problem all day, and had just had a 'Eureka!' moment, where all the faulty reasoning and wrong turns seemed worth it to get to this point.

My anxiety lifted along with my psychotic fog. 'You know what, Beck?' I said. 'You haven't been very sympathetic.'

She peered over at me. 'I'm sick,' she said.

This lit my fuse.

'You're always sick, Beck—always. What's wrong this time?'

'I've got sinus pain.'

'So you can't comfort me because you've got a blocked nose?'
She gave me an evil look.

'Ohhh, isn't that sad,' I continued. 'Poor little Beck has got a blocked nose.'

Beck jolted, as if she'd received an electric shock, and shouted, 'Perhaps I would have given you a bit more sympathy, Luke, if you haven't had sat there crying *like a fucking girl*.'

And then it was on.

Let me interject here for a second, and state what is probably obvious — I was in the beginnings of my crystal-meth binge. I had been using for about a month. I had become a little preoccupied myself, with maybes, and apparently probable — to me, at least — theories, and possible subterfuge. By this stage, my mission — to investigate crystal meth — had almost been forgotten. This was supposed to be my daring comeback into journalism, my chance to prove the haters wrong. I was here to cut through the spin and the hearsay reportage, and to find out precisely why meth had made a comeback of its own — into my life, and into the lives of many others — and was wreaking such havoc. Even if it wasn't the sort of havoc that made the news, and it was nothing like the havoc on the anti-meth adverts, it was havoc, nonetheless. The average drug-user — the one who used ecstasy and stayed away from heroin — was finding profound new highs in a substance that few of us had ever tried ever before, let alone understood. I, for one, was too involved in my elaborate paranoia to realise that what I was taking now was crystal meth, and that what I had been taking for the past few years had been powdered meth. This fact had been obscured to me by another fact: I had started injecting drugs again for the first time since my brief heroin foray in 2007.

When I first took the crystallised variety of meth at Smithy's in early 2014, I had no idea I was taking something different, and

I wonder how many users were in the same boat. The fact that so many different substances are all referred to as 'meth' only adds to the confusion. I thought the reason it felt so much stronger was that I was injecting it again, but it wasn't that simple.

The key to understanding how crystal meth came to supersede powdered meth in Australia is in, as explored in previous chapters, the growth of the production and consumption of the former in South-East Asia. Figures from the Australian Crime Commission show that while there was a 15 per cent increase in domestic lab detections between 2010–11 and 2011–12, and a steady increase over the past ten years, this figure did not compare to the enormous increase in international imports. And what was being imported was either crystal meth (which until very recently was almost certainly not being made here) or much more potent varieties of powdered meth.

The statistics on border detections tell a large part of Australia's crystal-meth story. The peak year for border detections of amphetamines between 2003 and 2011 was just under 600 detections in 2006–07 (years are counted in financial years), equalling about the same in kilograms. During many of the years throughout the 2000s, border amphetamine detections were at near negligible levels; for the year 2010–11, less than 100 kilograms were detected, and in 2011–12 there were about 300 kilograms discovered, relating to 1000 detections (then the highest number of detections on record).

Then, in 2012–13, the number rose to 1,999 detections. Yes, you did read that correctly, and it meant that the amount of meth being smuggled into our country increased by about 700 per cent, in terms of weight, from 2010 to 2013. The 2012–13 record high was eclipsed a year later, in 2013–14, by the new record of 2,367 detections.

As a result of the sharp increase in the amount of high-purity meth coming across the border, meth's purity in Australia saw a rise from an annual average of 21 per cent in 2009 to 64 per cent in 2013. In Victoria, the purity of meth rose from about 20 per cent in 2010–11 to more than 75 per cent in 2012–13. All in all, in the decade since 2004, the purity of methamphetamine (ice and speed) in Australia has generally increased, ranging between a median of 4.4 per cent and 76 per cent. The Victorian police — whose state records the highest purity — have labelled this a major factor in the meth problem: higher purity makes the drug more addictive.

And it wasn't just more pure; there was also more of it.

The reported use of powdered methamphetamine fell significantly between 2010 and 2013, but the reported use of crystal meth — what we by now knew as ice — more than doubled. People were also using ice more frequently, with many people using it daily or weekly. First, the number of methamphetamine users who prefer ice to other types of methamphetamine doubled from 27 per cent in 2007, and 22 per cent in 2010, to 50 per cent in 2013. The proportion of people using it at least weekly grew from 9.3 per cent in 2010 to 15.5 per cent in 2013. There was a corresponding increase in people seeking treatment at drug and alcohol clinics. The proportion of treatment 'episodes' where methamphetamine was the principal drug of concern doubled from 7 per cent in 2009–10 to 14 per cent in 2012–13.

The 2013–14 Australian Customs and Border Protection Service Annual Report shows crystal-meth detections by kilogram at our border. And when I say border, I should explain that crystal meth is mainly found amid the letters and parcels coming in via international post. According to data from the Australian Customs and Border Protection Service, 86 per cent of all crystal meth is coming via the parcel post, with another 9.5 per cent coming in via air cargo. According to data from the

ACC, no fewer than 49 countries were identified as countries of origin over the 2012–13 period. However, to simplify things somewhat: three territories account for 88 per cent of the total detections (when measured by weight). They are Hong Kong (96 detections, weighing a total of 224.1 kilograms); Thailand (43 detections, weighing a total of 313.9 kilograms); and China (8 detections weighing a total of 1224.6 kilograms). Therefore, based on figures of what is actually intercepted (2000 detections totaling 2,138.5 kilograms during that period), more than half of the amphetamines that are imported here are coming from the world's biggest nation.

Yep, China: the world's most populous nation is third behind the US and Mexico on the global meth pie chart, and is where most of our meth is coming from (this doesn't mean it's all being *made* in China, but it is certainly the major transit point). Indeed, meth is big business in China: confiscations of meth pills went up 1,500 per cent across the nation in the four-year period from 2008 to 2012. There is mounting evidence that the nation is actually supplying the cartels with precursors — that is, ephedrine and pseudoephedrine — which isn't surprising when you consider that the country is filled with, and surrounded by, ephedra plants.

According to UNODC, the average street price per gram of methamphetamine in China is A$105, whereas in Australia it is $500. Wholesale prices in Australia have been recorded as ranging from A$90,000 to A$325,000 per kilogram.

And to be even more specific: thanks to United Nations data, we know that most of the meth coming to Australia from China originates in Guangdong, a province of over 100 million people on the South China Sea.

To give you an idea of where the meth so many Australians are taking is being made, and just how engaged some of these southern China communities are in meth production and distribution, let me take you to a little Guangdong village called Boshe. Boshe is isolated, right on the coastline. It has no more than 1,700 households, and the last official estimate put the village population at approximately 14,000. Boshe isn't much to look at—in fact, it's like the worst of the old and new worlds deliberately came together on the marshy, sandy flatlands of the Southern Chinese coast to highlight what happens when a society fails. Boshe resembles some kind of mythic dystopia, with a mix of rural despair, urban decay, a few trees, abandoned buildings, cramped living, and a Technicolor dream-coat of plastic rubbish enmeshed in the soil just about everywhere you step. Amid this ghetto-come-junkyard—though it's not quite bleak enough to be classified a slum—if you were to walk through the mud, the pollution, and the litter, you would most likely notice an acidic, cat-piss-like odour that hits your nose like a bunch of blunt needles. The closer you look at the piles of garbage dumped around vacant housing lots, the more you notice the used glass flasks and other lab equipment, surrounded by pools of sludge.

Boshe, as it turns out, has in years gone by been one of the biggest meth producers in China, and probably the world. Guangdong police estimated that around 20 per cent of the town was involved in meth production in Boshe, and corruption went all the way to the top: the people running the meth trade in Boshe were government officials. Fourteen of them all up, and the local Communist Party secretary was in fact the local drug king pin, Cai Dongjia. Local police were in on it, too, colluding with local criminal groups to provide what seemed like a watertight and highly profitable illicit market. Today, there are even signs that read 'discarding of meth lab garbage here is forbidden'.

Chinese police knew what was happening in Boshe for a long time. In August 2013, police had tried to enter the village, but were met with roadblocks, people hurling abuse, and violent resistance. Peter Barefoot on Chinasmack.com writes that before the Thunder Drug Raid:

> As soon as the police entered the village, they'd be surrounded by the two to three hundred motorcycles in the village, with nail boards placed on the roads in the village, and rocks thrown from the top of buildings. Villagers would hold imitation firearms, even AK47s, homemade grenades, crossbows, and other deadly weapons.

The police retreated and re-evaluated the situation, deciding that they needed to go in better armed and better resourced — although few could have imagined just how well armed and resourced they would be when they finally returned a few months later. In China's coldest month, amid the drizzle and grey, 3,000 police surrounded Boshe. When the police got out of their vehicles, they were dressed in camouflage gear, and so the raids began. There were police vans on top of police vans, speedboats, and at least two helicopters accompanying the raid.

Police arrested 182 people, destroyed 77 methamphetamine labs, and a massive three tonnes of meth was seized along with 100 tonnes of meth ingredients. Cai Dongjia was the first to be captured. After completing the raid, the police said Boshe and the surrounding region were the source of a third of China's crystal-meth supply.

They later discovered that the village had become so polluted with chemicals for drug manufacturing that the groundwater could not be used for farming. Locals reported that a huge wealth gap had developed between the farmers in town and those involved in the drug trade. Indeed, entrepreneurialism and economic inequality could have a lot to answer for in explaining why China has become our biggest trading partner in both legal and illegal markets. Australia pays a lot for meth compared to our Asian neighbours. While China has increasingly advanced technology, it still has very low production and labour costs—big profits are to be made by making meth in poorer nations, and then selling them to high-income nations like Australia. Trafficking a highly addictive, highly pleasurable drug into a nation that is surrounded by some of the biggest meth-producing countries in the world must seem like a no-brainer to drug barons all over the world.

And we are not talking about one particular set of groups with names or brands, or any one particular country or region—in the transnational illicit-drug game, allegiances often only exist for a short time, and most of these 'groupings' are informal, fleeting, and very hard to track down.

With all this taken together, it is very tricky for our authorities to get a handle on the problem.

If there is one common fuel to this engine right around the globe, however, it is the bribing of high-level government officials in often weak, poorly resourced states that help get the drug cartels into gear. While we might know this is happening, stopping it is another thing altogether, especially when crime cartels are paying members of the government far more than they would be getting on their taxpayer-funded salary. In this way, poor and weak nations make the perfect hunting ground for criminal entrepreneurs to make it rich. And indeed, some of them are very rich—the illicit-drug trade makes up 1 per cent of the total global economy. The illicit-drug trade is the largest in value among global illicit commodities, at some US\$320 billion, according to the United Nations World Drug Report—an unwelcome, though arguably inevitable, consequence of an increasingly globalised economy.

Robert Mandel, who is the professor of international affairs at Lewis & Clark College in Portland, Oregon, argues in his book *Dark Logic: transnational criminal tactics and global security* that while Ronald Reagan started the 'global war on drugs' in 1985 with that very catch-cry — as well as with an allocation of hundreds of millions to the defence department to 'combat' the problem — the endeavour met with limited success:

> Any attempt to interdict global drug smuggling faces nearly insurmountable problems including (1) the eagerness of users/victims to imbibe, making them unlikely to press for prosecution of distributors; (2) reduced government monitoring of domestic activities due to economic liberalization and deregulation; (3) the proliferation of weak states which have remote areas conducive to drug growing and; (4) the scarcity of alternative sources of income for impoverished workers involved in the production of drugs.

And what I have told you about southern China is really just the cherry on top: it is unclear how much of the meth sent from Guangdong is being made in China, and how much of it is just distributed from there. If it is the latter, it is also not known precisely who Chinese criminals are linking with internationally. In many cases, it is likely to be groups in the jungles of the Golden Triangle — that infamous patch of jungle comprised of Myanmar, Vietnam, Laos, and Thailand where crystal meth is known to be made en masse. Much like the Mexican cartels, the Golden Triangle is likely going through an 'upgrade,' as a paper from Brookings Institute put it, and 'transforming from traditional drugs to new synthetic drugs, following demand of the international drug market'.

So our relationship with the illicit drug trade is 'complicated', and to make it even more so, today's problem region might be tomorrow's massive headache. The latest intelligence suggests parts of the Middle East and western Africa — regions usually associated with transit points for drugs—are now increasingly producing meth, particularly Iran and Nigeria. In fact, there is at least a 50 per cent chance that the gear my friends were selling was manufactured overseas. AFP Assistant Commissioner Ramzi Jabbour told the Victorian parliamentary committee at a hearing that: 'These very large seizures were being attempted to be imported into Australia, or in this case particularly Victoria, from overseas, and we allege by sophisticated organised criminal syndicates which have tentacles both in this country and reaching out through numerous countries overseas'. In many cases, crystal-meth users in Australia don't even go through their local dealer—they simply order from one of the many websites from which people can purchase meth and other drugs from overseas. While the notorious Silk Road site has closed down, many others have emerged in the space known as the 'Dark Web'.

The net result has not just been a stronger drug flooding our drug markets, but a significant global shift in drug use: according to 2013 data from UNODC, ATS were used, in 2011, at rates higher than any other drug class with the exception of cannabis. The number of cannabis users worldwide (on an annual basis) is estimated to be about 180 million, ATS users about 34 million, opiate users 16.5 million, and cocaine users about 17 million.

Today, we live not so much in a meth nation as a meth world: meth use is now an issue in most parts of the world, from the working classes of the United States to the middle classes of New Zealand, and from the shanty towns of South Africa to the increasingly affluent young people in Indonesia, the Philippines, Fiji, Thailand, and India. In Europe, the Czech Republic remains the focal point for the drug in the region, where it is called Pervitin. In Sweden, Finland, Slovakia, and Latvia, UNODC reports that amphetamines and methamphetamine users account for between 20 per cent and 60 per cent of those seeking drug abuse treatment. There are few nations around the world that remain untouched by meth.

After the argument with Beck that day, Smithy and I made up from our little incident a few hours earlier. Our physical altercation in 2011 (and our recovery from it) had actually strengthened our friendship—I think we both knew how difficult we could be. A little while earlier, I had thought he was orchestrating a cruel and vengeful plot; now we were the best of buddies again, with bong smoke consuming the space between us, and most sentences finishing with uncontrolled giggles. He had come back from Beck's, where he'd given her a small fix. She had, reportedly, lost her grimace, cured her cold, and was now vigorously washing rocks in her basin with her rock book next to her.

Smith had given me a tiny hit, too. It hadn't knocked my socks off, but it was enough to make me feel more energised: like a car that had been running on a low tank, but now had a bit in reserve. I felt calm—intensely calm—and knew that Smithy was a blood brother once again.

'That's it, the last of it,' he said, looking at me meaningfully. 'Y'know what that means?'

'We are both going to go clean and never use drugs again?'

'Hilarious—it means we have to go for a drive.'

'Where?'

'St Kilda.'

So we jumped in the car. We drove along what was in reality an uneventful freeway, but which felt, on this day, like the road to some of the greatest pleasures a man could ever know. We threw words around like confetti; Smithy talked about cricket, I talked about the way I got my job at triple j. Smithy said he had been texting Beck's oldest daughter for the past few months because it was 'important she had a parent right now', and as the wind blew around the car, and we smoked cigarette after cigarette, Smithy said, 'Is it just me, or do you smell like cat shit?'

We got to the dealer's house, and Smithy went to the door. After a while he came back, remarkably calm, and said, 'There's nobody fucking home, and he's not answering his phone.' It was warm inside the car, but I suspect Smithy, who was resting outside the car against the door, was feeling much warmer; he's an intolerable, catatonic, hot mess when he can't have drugs.

We asked a prostitute on the side of the road if we could pay her to find us some meth. She said her name was Celia, and agreed to help us out, but only if we gave her a cut.

'One of you need to come with me. Just one of you — if I bring two guys in he will freak out.'

I agreed to go, and so we walked silently together down the street, and the prostitute took me around the corner, then down a little side-alley, until we reached a set of white-brick apartments about three storeys high.

'It's not a houso block, by the way,' she said, smirking. 'It's a boarding-house, love. If you love freaks, you'll love these guys.'

From the front yard, we could see a 7-Eleven sign on the horizon, amid a row of oak trees. She knocked on the door.

'Who is it?' a grubby-sounding voice yelled.

'It's Celia, darl.'

'What do you want?'

'A bottle of chardonnay.'

A man opened the door. He was a tall, broad guy with short dark hair and dark skin, and he was wearing a large purple T-shirt and brown tracksuit pants. He had a mono-brow, and some of the hairs in it looked as long as my little finger.

He ushered us in. There were two other guys there — both men in their forties, old-timers with caps and tattoos — sharing a joint. The place was smaller on the inside that it looked from out. It was also musty, and there were barely any windows. There was a tiny lounge room, a small bedroom that barely fit one bed, and a kitchen—where everyone was standing—which was the biggest room in the unit.

'Who's this guy?'

'This is my friend, Luke,' Celia said. 'He wants two points.'

'Two points, hey?' he said, staring at me wide-eyed, his pupils swishing like two vibrating eggs.

'Luke, is it? Fucking let me tell you something, okay,' he said, eyes getting bigger and his movements looking almost comically self-righteous as he puffed out his chest. 'I am a fucking pharmacist, do you understand me?'

I nodded.

He thumped on his chest 'Me, I am a fucking chemist, the chemist, okay—I am the fucking chief, do you understand?'

Ignoring him, Celia flashed $200. 'Got those points, babe?'

'Here and here,' he said, passing them on to Celia, who immediately passed them to me. I looked at the bags of small clear crystals—innocuous, clean-looking—pretending that I knew what I was looking for.

'Sit down,' the chief said.

'No babe, I think he has to—'

'Sit down! In my culture, if somebody doesn't sit down, if they don't work a trade, if they are not polite to the chief, they get the *shaka*,' he said, raising his fist with his little finger and thumb raised on either side—what my generation would probably understand as the 'ridgey didge' symbol.

Celia was trying to hold back her laughter.

I pulled up a seat in the dining table. The chief pulled up a chair next to me and said 'But I am not going to give you the shaka. I am a *chemist*.'

It had been a long couple of days. Proving why white middle-class pencil-pushers should never, ever try to go ghetto, I said, with a tinge of sarcasm:

'Are you actually a chemist? I mean do you actually have a chemistry degree?'

The Chief ejected himself from his chair with a jolt, panting madly, walked over to the door, and slammed it shut.

'Nobody is fucking going anywhere, nobody leaves unless I say they can, and under my terms. Do you all fucking understand?'

## Chapter Eight

# Wheeling and dealing

MUCH TO THE disappointment of many of those I have met in my life, I *did* manage to survive that afternoon with the Chief, thanks to the quick-thinking Celia, who asked the Chief to get her something from his bedroom before leaning into me and whispering 'run'. We were out the door before the Chief realised we were gone. Two minutes later, I was safe: back in the car with Smithy, fielding all manner of questions about why it took so long and where we could get some syringes. I was glad we didn't have to regularly endure such trips to score. In fact, travelling nearly an hour to get crystal meth was a rarity for us — and pretty much everyone else — post-2011 in Australia. It isn't hard to find crystal meth once you start looking for it.

The Victorian branch of the Australian Medical Association told the Victorian parliamentary inquiry that 'the drug is exceptionally cheap and easy to obtain'. Indeed, Smithy's trips into town were very rare. To support both his habit and his own low-level dealing, he had multiple dealers to choose from — dealers who traded in both wholesale and retail. With this in mind, as well as the low cost of crystal meth, it should come as no surprise that even welfare recipients can inject the drug several times a day. Others—such as me—used less: a dose that can last many users up to twenty-four hours costs somewhere between $30 and $50.

From about 2011 onwards, if you were buying crystal meth in South Australia, you may well have bought it from a minion for an Outlaw Motorcycle Gang (OMCG); in Wangaratta, you may have bought it from a makeshift drug syndicate run by a former sports hero gone bad; or in Brisbane, you may have bought it from Patrick 'Ryan' McCann, a suburban real-estate agent who was earning as much as $100,000 a month in property commissions, but who, behind closed doors, was a daily drug-user, hiding silver bags of methamphetamine in his home.

And if you were in certain parts of Perth, the secret code to getting your gear was 'Hot Wheels'. To be more specific: you might have been told to go up to a paraplegic in a wheelchair and use a special code, after which he would reach down and pull a point or two out of his socks. Wheelchair-bound Ryan James Salton was arrested in July 2014 during a hospital visit. When he faced court, WA police alleged that they found four bags of methamphetamine hidden in socks in Salton's tracksuit pants, as well as a 'sweet puff' (crystal meth) pipe. Prior to the hospital incident, police had found the 33-year-old in bed next to a toiletry bag that contained his personal belongings as well as several drugs, at a house where Salton was believed to be living. It was also alleged that electronic scales, a gun, and a CCTV system that monitored access to the building were found at the house, as well as $5,000 cash hidden in a wheelchair. After he was charged, he was placed on bail, where it is alleged he committed further offences: police alleged they found him with hundreds of grams of methamphetamine in tablet and crystal form, almost $45,000 in cash, and a list of customers he had sold drugs to 'on tick'. Police would also allege that Salton's drug-dealer nickname was none other than 'Hot Wheels'.

Australia's meth dealers are an extremely diverse bunch. The ACC told the Victorian parliamentary inquiry that:

> No one criminal syndicate, type of crime group, or ethnicity-based group are dominant in the methamphetamine market in Victoria. Members of Outlaw Motorcycle Gangs (OMCGs), family groups, ethnic groups and entrepreneurial individuals working alone or in partnership are represented. The methylamphetamine market is sufficiently diverse and profitable to support a large number of competing and sometimes collaborating suppliers, at different levels of sophistication.

Later, a joint submission from six federal government agencies, including the Australian Crime Commission and the Australian Institute of Criminology, would tell the federal inquiry into crystal methamphetamine that:

> More than 60 per cent of Australia's highest risk criminal targets on the National Criminal Target List are known to be involved in the methylamphetamine market. Approximately 45 per cent of the highest risk criminal targets in the methylamphetamine market are characterised as OMCGs. The rest of the crystal meth dealing and manufacturing market remains then somewhat of a mystery.

This supports research by University of Queensland legal academic Andreas Schloenhardt, whose 2007 study found that within the methamphetamine drug market in Australia 'a changing mix of criminal elements is present, ranging from highly sophisticated and structured criminal organisations to individuals operating within small, local markets and friendship circles'. Other research from NDARC suggests that most meth users buy their meth off a friend, rather than a 'formal' drug dealer. Making in-roads into the problem of supply, particularly in the context of a rapidly expanding international market, has proven difficult for authorities; a legal database search shows meth-dealer convictions on any level are extremely rare.

I asked the ACC what the impact of the international trade had been on the local market. Their CEO Chris Dawson told me:

> There is no evidence that increases in the frequency and weight of methylamphetamine importations into Australia have led to a reduction in domestic production. What seems to have occurred is that both the level of domestic production and supply of methylamphetamine and the market share of imported (particularly crystal) methylamphetamine have increased.

Simultaneously, local manufacturers 'picked up their game' and began making higher-purity meth; it's probably only a matter of time before they start making crystal meth en masse. It would be a lucrative business — nationally, Australians are spending more than $7 billion each year on illicit drugs, according to research from the Bureau of Statistics. This is far more than our federal and state governments spend each year on law enforcement, treatment, and harm minimisation combined. That said, it's difficult to argue that spending more on law enforcement would make too much difference — as it stands, Australia's drug-dealer scene is messy, chaotic, disorganised, and very difficult to police. Alison Ritter from NDARC told me that she doesn't think organisations such as the Australian Federal Police have really started to unravel the big operators behind Australia's crystal-meth trade, unless 'they have people are currently embedded or working undercover, or perhaps they are collecting evidence — and in that case we might see some bigger convictions in years to come'.

What our federal authorities do seem to have worked out is that illicit-drug trafficking is closely linked to money laundering that is filtered through apparently legitimate businesses. In December 2012, the Australian Crime Commission Board approved the Eligo National Task Force, which it described as 'an Australian Crime Commission-led special investigation into the use of alternative remittance and Informal Value Transfer Systems by serious and organised crime … Eligo National Task Force is made up of the Australian Crime Commission, the Australian Transaction Reports and Analysis Centre (AUSTRAC) and the Australian Federal Police'.

The taskforce has made several significant drug busts, collecting tens of millions of dollars, and, for instance, leading a joint police operation in Tasmania and Queensland with transnational connections that in July 2014 led to the arrest of six men, including four members of the Rebels motorcycle club, on charges relating to the alleged trafficking, possession, and importation of more than 8 kilograms of amphetamine from the United Kingdom. The drugs were believed to have an estimated street value of at least $20 million. In a press release, Tasmania Police Assistant Commissioner Donna Adams said 'Criminal entities including OMCGs are developing in sophistication. This is why collaborative efforts by law enforcement agencies are an important element in staying ahead of the game'. In November 2014, the Serious and Organised Crime Branch of South Australia Police launched Operation Jackknife and nabbed an Adelaide crime group distributing methamphetamine from Malaysia to South Australia and Singapore. Police alleged the ringleaders of the importation in South Australia were the Rebels and Finks bikie gangs.

However, contrary to what some may be led to believe, bikies have not been involved in most of the nation's high-profile meth-dealing arrests. Australia's second-largest meth bust came in February 2013 after a single phone call to police from an anonymous source sparked a yearlong investigation that netted Australia's then-largest recorded crystal-meth seizure—585 kilograms worth an estimated $438 million.

In Philip K. Dick's 1977 science-fiction masterpiece *A Scanner Darkly*—set in the not-too-distant future, in a futuristic, totalitarian society—America has lost the war against drugs, and paranoia and big corporations reign. Law enforcement has been completely privatised, and undercover detective Bob Arctor is working with a group of small-time drug users trying to reach the big distributors of a brain-damaging drug called Substance D. Bob starts to take the drug, and begins to lose his mind. His reality shatters into a psychotic matrix, and his identity begins to split in two.

Substance D, the drug in Dick's novel, is described as being quite amphetamine-like. Dick himself was an enthusiastic speed-user at various points in his life: by 1971, he was ingesting a whopping 1,000 speed pills a week, along with plentiful tranquilisers. Dick wrote *A Scanner Darkly* after several years of firsthand experience with what he called the 'street scene' in the early 1970s.

In the novel, Arctor says that being addicted is like being sentient yet not alive: 'Seeing and even knowing, but not alive. Just looking out. Recognising but not being alive. A person can die and still go on. Sometimes what looks out at you from a person's eyes maybe died back in childhood.' Dick describes Arctor's thoughts on the drug thus: 'Someday, he thought, it'll be mandatory that we all sell the McDonald's hamburger as well as buy it; we'll sell it back and forth to each other forever from our living rooms. That way we won't even have to go outside.'

Dick's vision is grim, where the collusion of state-corporate power and drug addiction are intimately linked, and where the very ideals of individualism, freedom, and self-possession have not only reached their limits, but become perverse.

Bob Arctor seems to ache so badly from the lack of adventure and meaning in suburban culture that he descends into drug abuse to escape. Dick's novel was written at a time when the beatnik and hippie movements of the 1950s and 1960s had run their course. Drugs were used within these subcultures to attempt to expand consciousness, but by the 1970s they seemed to people like Dick to be ways of confusing reality for users, so that otherwise revolutionary thinkers were too incoherent to dissent in any meaningful way. Rather than find a way to improve or progress an over-sterilised, over-controlled suburban environment, Bob is so self-focused that he chooses simply to alter his perception of it.

On describing the nihilism of suburban drug addicts, Arctor said: 'They wanted to have a good time, but they were like children playing in the street; they could see one after another of them being killed—run over, maimed, destroyed—but they continued to play anyhow.'

There is no apparent choice of a more interesting, fulfilling life. The people Bob meets live in a haze of drug use, and he never gets close to the mysterious drug syndicate, while the corporation's quest to defeat it seems like an incredibly superficial response to an environment which lends itself so easily to drug addiction. In other words, catching the syndicate—which we get the sense may not even exist—seems fruitless when the demand to deal and use the drug is a cogent response to a culture that has bred this kind of appetite for drugs in the first place.

If you added youth unemployment to Dick's unstable societal mix, you'd be getting close to a remarkable turn of events that took place in Wangaratta, three hours from Melbourne. In 1999, the town of 17,000 looked like it might have a new sporting hero. Eighteen-year-old Aaron Shane Dalton—tall and strong, with dark brown hair—was restless and rebellious in school, but seemed to have found the right outlet for all his energy: cycling. His father, an abattoir manager and part of a well-respected family in the area, was delighted when his son ditched his pot habit for a sport that required endurance, patience, power, and tactical nous. So delighted was his father, in fact, that he organised for his son to be trained by former Olympic gold medallist Dean Woods. Dalton trained like a demon under Woods; he trained at the Victorian Institute of Sport, and eventually became one of the top ten riders of his age group in Australia. Ultimately, though, like many young men before him, Dalton found that even his best wasn't enough: he wanted to turn professional, and to do that he almost certainly needed to get a scholarship at the Australian Institute of Sport. Dalton didn't make the cut. He gave up on cycling and threw himself into drug taking, soon graduating to amphetamines. He began dealing meth, and, despite getting convicted twice—once in 2006 and again in 2009—he masterminded one of the most sophisticated drug syndicates regional Australia had ever seen. Dalton discovered an ice manufacturer in Grafton, in country New South Wales, and then started recruiting distributors, drivers, 'logistics' people, and heavies. Dalton cashed in at the right time—ice was now on the market, and he found plenty of dealers with recurring customers around Shepparton, Wodonga, Yarrawonga, Myrtleford, Corowa, Rutherglen, and Wangaratta. In less than eighteen months, the syndicate—and especially Dalton—was raking in millions. His drivers were known to collect up to $250,000 worth of ice at a time from Grafton. In some cases, they would pick up the gear and then hire expensive hotel rooms in Albury, where they would weigh and package the drug, sometimes burying it in the ground near the hotel to store it for future use. Dalton found a few locals who were desperate to be liked and who desperately wanted friends, including 26-year-old Jai Montgomery, who had a missing limb, and 26-year-old Kruchan Chandler, who had played semi-professional football before a devastating knee injury destroyed his career. Dalton was extremely professional and cautious in his operation. Computer-generated documents were used, but there were protocols for destruction of written materials. When a distributor or driver joined the network, they were given a four-page instruction letter on how to conduct themselves in public. The document instructed that the syndicate was in the 'business of making money, not power-tripping or disrespecting customers', and any complaints would be investigated. 'This is how serious we are about the professionalism of our services which you require.'

Customers were given code words to use on phones when placing orders: 'catch up for a coffee' translated into 0.1 of a gram of ice, and 'catch up for a bourbon' meant one gram. The instructions included a warning that there would be harsh consequences for anyone who acted unprofessionally or dared commit the 'vile act' of going to the police. Dalton ruled with an iron fist: he hired 24-year-old Muay Thai fighter Dean Griggs as the syndicate's tough guy. Over time, a young butcher was shot at his home in a busy residential street, two homes were firebombed as children slept inside, and cars were set alight. Recovering drug debts and maintaining territory was a vicious process, and often involved weapons. If a person left the syndicate, Griggs was known to interrogate them violently in their home.

Wangaratta Police launched Operation Juliet and eventually caught up with Dalton, who—much to the relief of his own family—was arrested in September 2012. The full extent of his syndicate's operations were laid out in court nearly two years later, and, in July 2014, he was sentenced to a maximum of nine years in jail after pleading guilty to trafficking a commercial quantity of methamphetamine—known as ice—and ecstasy, as well as recklessly causing serious injury, reckless conduct endangering a person, false imprisonment, and arson. Eight others were charged, and another four, including Dalton's brother and ex-girlfriend, would later be convicted.

During the trial, Aaron's father Shane Dalton told the court that he was relieved when his son was arrested: 'We didn't know what was going to happen. At least if he was in jail, we knew he was going to be safe.' He said that he saw his son slip into the problem in mid-2012, after his partner and young daughter left him.

Fleeting, opportunistic, and surprisingly sophisticated: Australia's meth scene was creating instant criminals—often with little or no prior criminal history—who wanted a slice of the action. It's not surprising that many people—often youngish men—would be attracted to the idea of being a drug dealer in contemporary society. Drug dealing is one of the few vocations that crosses over between gangster street cred and celebrity, creating a kind of buoyant masculine glamour that can be either a consolation for failure in the mainstream or a suitable alternative to the blisters, bad backs, and slow-burn money-making of most working-class jobs and trades. For others, it might simply be a way of ensuring the phone is always ringing.

Smithy, I often noticed, charged people for drugs based on how sexually attractive he found them—which in my case meant I didn't get free drugs for standing there looking pretty, like many of the girls who came to the house did. However, when I first moved in, he came up to me one day when I was in the kitchen and whispered 'I'll offer you the same deal I offered Beck: you can give money for a hit or you can give me a blow job.'

Beck later denied that this was the set-up, suggesting Smithy might have been joking about the offer, although 'you can never be 100 per cent sure'.

Dodgy deals aside, I reckon we live in a society that not only expects us to fulfil our duty, but also wants us to discover what our duty is. We must find our own reference for meaning. Many of us long to find it in our daily lives, and eventually we ask ourselves: 'Can I work hard enough to dream?'

For Smithy, his casual drug dealing had started again, believe it or not, after Beck gave birth to their twin boys in 2009. Beck had fallen pregnant twice before in the first two years they were together, and terminated both pregnancies. Smithy had told her he was not interested in having children because he wanted to keep partying for the rest of his life, and didn't want the responsibility or financial burden of having kids.

After the birth, Beck went to work in the factory in Dandenong, and found the work a nice break from crying babies and the sight of her lounge-room walls. However, after hour upon hour of screwing together light globes and putting them inside little boxes, she found herself dreading work so much that she was having painful anxiety attacks. She resigned at the six-week mark, and Smithy took this as a serious, disappointing, but not altogether surprising broken promise. He now believed that not only had Beck deliberately fallen pregnant, but he was also faced with the prospect of working all week to feed his children and pay his rent, without a drug-fuelled 'Smithy Saturday' to look forward to. This was nothing short of a prison life, surely, though there was one thing he hadn't counted on: Smithy bonded with those beautiful little boys like a fish does with water, and he quite liked his new life. Nonetheless, he pressed Beck to make money, and she used her encyclopaedic knowledge of welfare law to good effect for a little while, but eventually she ran out of tricks. So Smithy started dealing pot. He'd buy it in bulk—on tick—sell it, smoke it, and then repay the wholesaler with his revenue—meaning all 'profit' went up in smoke. This non-profit, consignment model of small-time retail drug dealing was also readily applied when he started selling meth to his friends.

Like so many other young, small-time drug dealers, Smithy and Beck both had parents who never used drugs and were never involved in crime. They saw their parents work day after day, often for relatively long hours, without much pleasure or glory—at least not that they could see. And they grew up to find that getting meaningful employment was far harder for them, and required far more commitment and training—and for what? To spend all their money on a rental, or on a mortgage that required an average working-class person to work two jobs and eat Vegemite sandwiches for dinner every second night? Beck had an easier time applying her brains to mastering Centrelink than she did packing boxes. Smithy could have gone out to work as a labourer and earned $120 a day, or he could sit at home taking drugs, and selling them among his friends, for roughly the same result. I guess you could call it an underclass rebellion: a group of people who aspired to less of the material and career goals they'd seen their lower-middle-class parents struggle to attain. Meth use was a way of living in the moment and rejecting the stoic, disciplined lives of their parents. Instead, this was a group who thought hedonism and fun were the appropriate ways to live their lives—all part of their defiance against the expectations they work in arduous jobs like labouring or aged care.

I met other small-time drug dealers while I was living at Smithy's: three to be precise. There was 'Tall'—a 45-year-old former refrigerator repairman who I think meant well, but whose poor social skills meant he was bound for a lonely life. There was 'Short'—a young Italian-looking dude from the suburbs who tried to hide his tiny frame and highly sensitive personality with Adidas-style gangster wear. And there was 'Skinny'—a willowy, dark-haired former carpenter who walked in one day to see us watching netball on Foxtel and said 'Oh, netball. I used to play mixed netball down Knox way. Good on you, mate, good on you'.

All three seemed to come over to Smithy's at about the same rate. Tall would sometimes stay to socialise, and one day he said he'd found something he thought would be of particular interest to me.

'This will blow your mind, mate, blow your mind. Have you ever heard of Agenda 21?'

He played me a video on his iPad. The video was of a former South Australian Independent MP called Anne Bressington speaking on a podium at some unnamed event at the Adelaide Convention Centre. Bressington explained that 'the words of Agenda 21 were never meant to be spoken'. She said it had been created by a secret group called the Club of Rome, which invented a number of 'imaginary dangers' like global warming and water shortages as a way of creating globalisation. Australia, in turn, brought in a new economic order, leaving Australia short of technology, a manufacturing base, and jobs.

Tall stood over my shoulder watching it, nodding his head in agreement, and then shaking his head when he thought through the implications.

Agenda 21 is — in case you are wondering — a real thing: a non-binding, voluntarily implemented action plan of the UN with regard to sustainable development. For conspiracy theorists, it is part of a secret global agenda to depopulate the earth.

'We are constantly having our rights impinged upon,' Tall said after we'd watched the video. 'I can never make a profit from work, I can never get ahead, I can't afford a house, and it's all because of Agenda 21 — it's all because of the carbon tax.'

I explained that the carbon tax had been abolished, and oddly that seemed to be just a 24-hour obsession; Tall never mentioned Agenda 21 again. Instead, he began to focus his attention on Short, to whom he had given an amount of crystal meth to sell on consignment. Then — apparently long before the date when Short was supposed to return the profit — Tall started demanding the money back. Smithy told me this was because Tall was in the habit of injecting at our place, and then going around the corner to the oldest building in town—the Pakenham Hotel—and blowing all his money on the pokies. When Short was unable to return the funds on time, conflict ensued. Tall spent hours in our garage, fuelled up on meth, threatening to kill Short: 'If only I could find where he lives,' he would say, and then he'd put on his reading glasses and spend hours trawling through the White Pages online, Google maps, and various other websites from which he was convinced he'd be able to learn Short's whereabouts because he had his phone number. Eventually, he settled on sending threatening text messages.

Tall, Short, and Skinny all knew I was writing a book, so they were very, and understandably, reluctant to give me any information about who they sourced their drugs from, how they did their business, or how the drug-supply hierarchy worked. However, one did introduce me to one guy—I won't give too much away about him other than to say he worked for a major Melbourne underworld figure a few years back, and he had a number of contacts. One of his 'cooks' told me that home-made meth—the world's most powerful stimulant drug—can be made in our sinks, in our garages, and in our cars by shaking a Coke bottle containing some ingredients that have been blended in a food processor.

Towards the end of *A Scanner Darkly*, a character who appears fleetingly throughout the book is endlessly antagonised by imaginary bugs he sees all over himself, the floor, and his dog. Driven mad by his abuse of Substance D, he apparently decides to end his life by drinking and sleeping pills. He goes to bed inexplicably clutching a copy of Ayn Rand's *The Fountainhead* while a creature with many eyes all over it, wearing ultra-modern, expensive-looking clothing, rose eight feet high with a scroll to read all his sins. We are told this is going to take a hundred thousand years. Dick writes:

> Fixing its many compound eyes on him, the creature from between dimensions said, 'We are no longer in the mundane universe. Lower-plane categories of material existence such as "space" and "time" no longer apply to you. You have been elevated to the transcendent realm. Your sins will be read to you ceaselessly, in shifts, throughout eternity. The list will never end.' Know your dealer, Charles Freck thought, and wished he could take back the last half-hour of his life. A thousand years later he was still lying there on his bed with the Ayn Rand book … listening to them read his sins to him.

It is not precisely clear what Dick was intending to convey by placing Rand's book in this scene. Rand was a supporter of egoism and laissez-faire capitalism, and *The Fountainhead* is about one man's choice to live in obscurity to maintain his independence and integrity. Rand's philosophy was called 'Objectivism' — she described its essence as 'the concept of man as a heroic being, with his own happiness as the moral purpose of his life, with productive achievement as his noblest activity, and reason as his only absolute'. Rand's ideas would later influence a whole generation of libertarians; free marketeers who emphasised the importance of autonomy and individual choice without state or collectivist interference.

There is something to be said here about the connection between meth production and individualism; a person who makes their own meth — particularly an addict who uses their own products — is economically autonomous. The meth producer who works for his or her own self is atomised, has happiness as their central goal, is isolated, and is highly self-sufficient. They do not concern themselves with social expectations or what other people think. It makes me wonder: are they not a warped result of Ayn Rand's dream?

And as a result of the actions of these autonomous producers, clandestine lab detections — while not rising as quickly as importations of meth — have increased rapidly since 2009, doubling across the last decade. There were 314 detected nationally in 2002; 356 in 2007–08; 449 in 2008–09; 694 in 2009–10; and 744 in 2013–14. Queensland had a particularly monstrous rise: from 121 in 2007–08 to 379 over the 2011–12 period, before dropping back slightly to 340 in 2013–14.

That's an awful lot of toxic waste, cat-piss odours, and empty brake-fluid containers filling up Australian suburbs. And Australian suburbs are exactly where the police are finding this new wave of meth production. During 2011–12 and 2012–13, 68.2 per cent of clandestine laboratories were located in residential areas, followed by those in vehicles (9 per cent), commercial or industrial areas (8.9 per cent), public places (3.8 per cent), rural areas (2.2 per cent), and other places (7.9 per cent). However, unlike the big industrial-scale labs shown in *Breaking Bad* (which *do* exist all over Mexico and parts of South-East Asia) between 2011–12 and 2012–13 in Australia, the majority of detected clandestine laboratories were individual and addict-based (58.8 per cent), whereas others were small-scale labs (23.5 per cent), medium-sized labs (9.7 per cent) and industrial-scale labs (8 per cent), the latter of which had seen an increase from 2.7 per cent in 2011–12. Notable detections included a massive drug factory in Hume and another in South Australia, at a property at Walker Flat, where a drug lab was found in a shack on the banks of the Murray. Two Gold Coast men were jailed for their involvement in one of the most sophisticated 'factory style' meth labs ever seen in Australia: Dane Marriott, thirty-nine, and Matthew Smith, thirty-one, who were arrested after police raided their 'resort-style' property nestled in the Currumbin Valley back in June 2011.

The increase can be explained by simple supply and demand. However, the rise in individual labs also shows how relatively easy it is for untrained people to learn how to make meth. The method can found on the internet, and that is often where people are buying the ingredients as well. According to the Victorian parliamentary inquiry paper:

> The process of manufacturing methamphetamine using ephedrine and pseudoephedrine is not difficult. Extracting the precursor involves simply soaking the tablets in methylated spirits, decanting or filtering to remove sediment, and then evaporating the solvent, leaving the precursor.

Addict-based labs are also very difficult to police; the amount of resources used to find one single addict-lab may not be worth the effort. And even if the police *do* find one, it won't take long before another addict — perhaps in the same suburb, or even the same street — is going to learn how to do the same. All of this is in palpable contrast to other heavy drugs like heroin or cocaine, which need entire agricultural fields to grow. And while it has become far more difficult to get pseudoephedrine-based medications from chemists, it is thought that most addict-based labs are still using these medications to make their gear. Jason Ferris, who is a Senior Research Fellow at the Institute for Social Science Research (ISSR) at The University of Queensland, told me that all you need as base ingredients to make an entire gram of meth is in just two packets of Sudafed.

While there is now more potent meth on the market — that is, the crystallised form — all forms of methamphetamine are manufactured the same way. The form in which the end product is sold simply depends on how far the manufacturers extend the crystallisation process.

Now to an extremely important point, which is crucial to

understanding why meth has risen again as a problem in Australia in the last five years (this being in addition to the growth of South-East Asian production). In 2010, it came to the attention of police that a new, simple method for making powdered meth had been discovered and was being used widely—the 'shake and bake' method that allowed individual users to make meth quickly by shaking ingredients together in a plastic bottle

The 'shake and bake' method is a variation on the more traditional 'Nazi' method (which was indeed used extensively by the Nazis, and then by OMCGs in the early 1970s). This method retains the majority of crystal meth's traditional ingredients (pseudoephedrine, lithium, Coleman fuel, hydrochloric acid, etc.), but rather than using glassware and an open flame, they're mixed by shaking them all together in a regular plastic bottle with water. Nobody is sure who started this method, but it quickly spread from the United States to Australia. The entire process takes less than fifteen minutes, and is fast becoming the method of choice for ten of thousands of meth-producing addicts, creating a phenomenon known as rolling meth-labs: transportable laboratories which are often found in cars, hotel rooms, or rented properties. The end result is not as potent as crystal meth by any stretch of the imagination, however the ease with which it is made is clearly an issue for authorities who are understandably finding such vast, individualised production difficult to police.

One user, Helen, told me she makes her own meth using this home-made method. 'I guess anybody can make it, but making good stuff is hard,' she told me. 'I like to use a lot, so that's why I make my own batch.'

'How did you learn how to make it?'

'From a friend,' she said, going on to explain the process of making meth via the 'shake and bake' method—for obvious reasons, I will provide a mere skeleton view of what she told me.

'The first step involves grinding everything in a food processor, and then you shake it all up in an empty Coke bottle using lithium from a battery,' she said. 'The main ingredients are over-the-counter cold remedies. I know people who case big warehouses for this stuff, but most of the time I don't need it, because with a few packets I can make about three grams in a few hours.'

There are plenty of strange places where meth labs have been spotted: Melbourne police officers once discovered people cooking crystal meth and selling it from a van in a park, as if it were an ice-cream truck. In Bundaberg, a car was pulled over with smoke rolling out of its windows — the driver was making meth as he drove. At other times, it has been found in bathrooms, car boots, caravan parks, and even retirement homes. Hotel rooms can be the perfect place to make the substance, particularly when booked under false or no ID.

Drug manufacturers more generally seem to favour rented properties, so they don't have to carry the liability of a property that has become so infested with toxic smoke that it seeps poison out of the walls for months, even after a lab has been removed and the area has been professionally cleaned. First National Real Estate in Queensland even held two specific information sessions at its recent national Property Management Conference to ensure its property managers are fully equipped, both to identify and effectively manage their response to the rise of meth labs.

And in Australia, meth-lab cleaning is becoming a fast-growing industry. In 2011, the Meth Lab Clean-up Conference and mini trade-show, held on the Gold Coast, drew 150 delegates. Other exhibiters at the conference included Real Estate Dynamics, Veda, and AON, who have recently included cover of up to $10,000 for illegal drug production in their landlord insurance. Jena Dyco International, the leading Australasian trainer in carpet and upholstery cleaning and restoration, announced the addition of a new course to their scope aimed at teaching restorers how to clean-up and remediate illegal drug labs.

I spoke with Jenny Boymal from Jena Dyco, who said they had noticed a spike in the number of meth-lab cleaning inquiries from around 2010 onward.

'Government departments didn't know about it, nobody knew much about it, we actually had to contact a forensic scientist in New Zealand about it, and we developed the course as a result. It's not okay to say, "I have been cooking meth in this property—I'm going to paint the walls and she'll be right", because it won't be fine. It will seep right through the paint in many circumstances,' Jenny told me. She also explained just how toxic the stuff I had been injecting straight into my veins could be—or, at least, how toxic the production process is.

'The first thing we do is test for mercury and lead … what happens is that the smoke from the chemical process means these substances are in the wall, so if we find mercury and lead we need to more than just a surface clean; if you just do a surface clean then these substances will simply start seeping out every couple of months. If people live in this environment they often come down with colds. We know of one cleaning company that didn't use masks going in and they all came down with excruciating headaches after inspecting a meth-lab scene,' she said. 'Our cleaners usually go in with respirators, Tyvec suits, shoe coverings, gloves, and eye goggles.'

Each kilogram of meth manufactured creates 10 kilograms of waste. Ammonia and hydrogen chloride are both corrosive gases that will affect the eyes and respiratory tract, with damage increasing with concentration, and in a worst-case scenario, the result is pulmonary oedema and death. Currently, there are only state guidelines for meth clean-ups, and there is no obligation for landlords or prior owners to tell new tenants or purchasers that the property was used as a meth lab—a fact that has led to some calls for national disclosure laws.

Making meth is dangerous work. Royal Perth Hospital alone has treated at least 50 patients in the past five years for burns linked to methamphetamine manufacturing. It seems being a meth chemist can be dangerous and messy as well as lucrative.

Aaron Dalton's father told Fairfax media in May 2014 that he had watched his son transform during his two years in Port Phillip Prison. Aaron went from constantly talking of 'getting people back' to telling his father how bad ice was and what it was doing to people. Dalton is now studying behavioural science. Meanwhile, with Dalton behind bars, Wangaratta thought the worst of the crystal storm was behind them. History was, however, determined to tell a different story. Just a few months after Dalton's syndicate were dismantled, a new, highly sophisticated syndicate sprang up in the town. A few months after Dalton was put in jail, another gang — this time an OMCG — started selling meth in town, and police again went to work, making more arrests and seizing $100,000 of dollars worth of the drug

And as for 'Hot Wheels'? He was sentenced to eight years jail for drug trafficking on 19 December 2014. The 33-year-old Ryan Salton appeared in a hospital bed for his trial, in which Judge Anthony Serrick rejected any notion of lenience in his sentence because the paraplegic had a history of drug and firearm convictions.

## Chapter Nine

# Understanding the lure of crystal meth

THIS IS A surprisingly difficult sentence to write, but here goes: meth has a good side. It is a sentence I have to write, though, because if I am going to tell the story of meth, I have to tell you about all the fun times that I and others have had, and continue to have, on the world's most powerful stimulant.

I spoke with a number of users from different states in Australia, and from different walks of life, about their experience of meth, and each of them said very similar things about its positive qualities. When I asked one user (who wanted to remain anonymous) about meth's good side, he said it makes him feel 'giddy, like I'm in love' and as if every single cell in his brain 'is more alive than ever before, more awake, more happy than ever before. I feel like the most entertaining, edgy, cool fucker whoever did live'.

One woman who works a 9–5 office job and maintains a marriage and three kids in the western suburbs of Sydney reported that, for her, taking meth feels like 'getting something done; I feel this immense sense of pride, as if I'm the smartest and most accomplished person … I feel flawless, and that I haven't made a single mistake in my whole life'.

If we take her line of reasoning a little further, we could arrive at the following: 'You can do anything and be anything you want in life with just a sprinkle of meth'. From my experience, I would say this is true, provided you don't want it done particularly well, and provided that nobody rudely taps you on the shoulder to say 'it's all in your fucking head' — which is unlikely to occur if you surround yourself with other meth users.

Using crystal meth makes it difficult to tell the difference between what is real and what is not. It enables you to construct a fantasy that what other people (who, in reality, are all as self-centred as each other) do and think revolves around you and how good you are. Meth psychosis and its self-centred excesses are really just a more extreme version of the individual narcissism that meth creates.

After the initial rush, meth users are often enraptured by fantasies that they experience as either real, imminently real, or a hidden truth that they have finally discovered. The fantasy world creates the impression of a new, higher, more authentic, and ultimately more satisfying form of meaning. A shot of meth effectively goes straight to the brain, where it quickly forms a bubble cushioning you from the banality of the here-and-now, as well as from the failures and shortcomings of your past life and self. The consequence is that users tend to think of themselves as much more successful than their actual lives would suggest. Crystal meth allows you to become pleasantly confused about who you are, and these daydreams of imminent achievement become so real that they are instantly incorporated into your definition of self. The drug allows the construction of a new life narrative — a simplistic, victorious mythology, in which you are not only as beautiful, strong, successful, and popular as you can possibly be, but also that you are more beautiful, stronger, more successful, and more popular than anybody else in the room.

This process of believing your own delusions is what I call

being in the world of 'Fantasia'. I'm not talking about psychosis, or crazy out-there ideas like being able to fly or being a foot taller than you really are; Fantasia is when a waking fantasy means you think you have achieved your ego ideal. It's almost as if you are a kite, and your ego swells roughly to the level of how high you are flying.

Molly Andrews writes in her book *Narrative Imagination and Everyday Life*: 'We know that the not-real might also be the not-yet-real, and that that which is real is never a static category … The real and not-real are not then polar opposites.'

Once you come out of Fantasia, you are presented with a chance to reach genuine revelation — or, at least, it seems that way. It seems, in fact, as if you have a clean slate. You have to pick up the pieces, to find a way to work out what is actually true: where imagination ends and reality begins.

My experience of Fantasia taught me that the ways in which we construct our selves and our egos are built equally on our fantasies of ourselves, our interpretation of the past, and our expectations of the future. Much of our life is given meaning through mythology, fantasy, and imagination, such as, for example, the 'fantasy' of currency's value, the 'fantasy' of property rights, of the need for fixed working hours, the 'fantasy' of the ideal self in a media- and marketing-saturated world. I hope I haven't lost you here: please allow me to explain.

Prior to moving into Smithy's house, I had been living in Darlinghurst, Sydney. I really disliked the city, and I disliked the Oxford Street strip particularly. But when I reflected upon this after coming out of a Fantasia trip, I felt it had become clear to me that it was a place where people were trapped in their own imaginations. In particular, the imagined value of property, both to own and rent, meant people worked long hours in jobs which were not very fun, sacrificing weekends, weeknights, and treating their minds like they were working in a nineteenth-century factory. Why? As far as I could tell, the professional middle classes of inner Sydney believed themselves to be in the throes of an imaginary social hierarchy, a bit like professional tennis players who play each week to improve their ranking. Many of those at the upper end of the scale longed to be in the elite—which meant owning a house that they and our society recognised as being of high value, and working in a job that, while not enjoyable, placed them at the top of an invisible ranking. Eventually, everything about the experience led me to believe that the conventions of bourgeois life were a charade; from the homogenised dress code and mannered passive-aggression of it all to the fact that people worked unnecessarily long hours to pay off ridiculously over-inflated mortgages.

As a gay man, I noticed that virtually all the gay men living around Darlinghurst pretty much looked the same and many, including myself, spent hours in the gym after work to maintain muscular bodies so they could feel 'in the game' or even that they were 'winning the game'—even though, for the most part, nobody spoke a word to each other in the gym. Everyone seemed very self-absorbed, and it was difficult to believe they really cared about anyone else. This was a city where homosexuality was embraced, and yet some homosexuals living within it had found their way into another type of oppression—the prison of the modern citizen. I was living in the gayest area in town, yet there was no sense of community. Then came the Gay and Lesbian Mardi Gras, which was sponsored by a bank that year, and had what seemed to be a majority of corporate floats—corporations, of course, being the essential beneficiaries of this type of society. Now here's the bit where I admit to something really unpleasant about myself as well: there were many times when I was strolling through the streets of Sydney—with its franchise-filled shopping strips and gay men wearing gangsta-black basketball tops—that I began to fantasise about using meth. Fantasise perhaps isn't even the right word — crave, water at the mouth. Similarly, one of Chuck Palahniuk's character in his novel *Survivor* notes that, 'You realise that people take drugs because it's the only real personal adventure left to them in their time-constrained, law-and-order, property-lined world. It's only in drugs or death we'll see anything new, and death is just too controlling.'

Despite meth's atomising, individualising effects, there is no doubt that drugs also bring people together. One of the major appeals of crystal meth, for me, remained the intimacy and affiliation of using with others. We had sleepless nights and endless private jokes. There is a certain ritualistic spirituality to preparing and injecting drugs. When I shot up, I felt as if I was also shooting down the invisible walls and hierarchies that divide us. I used to love going to Smithy's room with a few of his straight mates, shutting the door, getting the spoons out, boiling water, and mixing the gear — knowing that not only would I get high, but that we would all share in it together, and share that bond for the rest of our lives. (Although, to be honest, there are few things more awkward than meeting a former drug buddy when you're no longer using. You generally find that not only do you have nothing in common with them, but that you don't particularly like them.) I would get excited when I heard the kettle boil at 2.00am, knowing Smithy didn't drink coffee or tea. If I saw a few ratbags going into a room, the door shutting behind them, it was very hard not to gently knock and ask if I could join them. Injections often took place just after midnight — my favourite time — and I loved living in a house that was often a buzz of activity right through the night. There were always people hovering around, feeling that weird mix of trepidation and elation at the prospect of letting a grubby little junkie inject them with a sharp, fresh needle. After taking meth, any social anxiety or awkwardness would be instantly lifted. My confidence would skyrocket, and at times I would even feel superior to those who were too afraid to use syringes — it seems that as one hierarchy disappears, another appears in its place.

All things considered, though, it is perfectly legitimate to ask whether meth experiences such as these are genuinely cathartic, or whether they are, in fact, just re-opening old wounds (or creating new ones). Does drug use expand your consciousness, or shrink it? One group of people who had to ask real questions about themselves and the world because of their experience with drugs was the infamous American Beatniks: by the mid-1940s Beat-Generation writers Jack Kerouac, William Burroughs, and Allen Ginsberg were sharing a drab apartment on 115th Street on the west side of New York. Searching for a new type of experience and creative flow, one that was free of restrictive thinking, they began to experiment, at first with Benzedrine (benzo) inhalers and pills.

Kerouac was a particular fan. He would write to Ginsberg saying that Benzedrine 'made me see a lot. The process of intensifying awareness naturally leads to an overflow of old notions and voila, new material wells up like water forming its proper level and makes itself evident at the brim of consciousness'. Kerouac loved to get on the gear and listen to jazz and bebop; he then tried to emulate the sounds in his writing.

Was Kerouac actually becoming more creative? Was it opening his mind? Or was he just becoming over-confident? Well, he *would* go on to write the poetically titled *On The Road* on a three-week benzo bender during which he barely slept a wink. There is no question that the Beat Generation enjoyed the glow from the golden age of amphetamines for both creative and social purposes.

And during my first six weeks on the drug, I can't deny I did a truckload of writing and had an enormous amount of fun while doing it. It helped me write creatively not simply because it enhanced my imagination, but also because it gave me confidence, and silenced that annoying writer-block-inducing voice that was forever telling me 'your work is shite'. Writing and meth seemed to be a very good combination. Meth might make you more creative, but that doesn't necessarily mean it will also increase the quality of your work; it is effective in producing original ideas, but they won't always favourably compare to the ideas that will come if you really apply yourself creatively, without drugs. Dopamine is not only characteristic of a psychotic, over-confident brain, but it also characterises a highly creative brain. While there was often very little that separated my experiences of psychosis and controlled creativity, in the end it was over-confidence and infantile delusion that won out.

Psychologist Nicole Lee believes there are six main forms of methamphetamine use — experimental, recreational, circumstantial, binge, regular use, and polydrug use — and has noted that dependence is more likely to be associated with regular use. But the demographics of who uses meth are also revealing. Writing in *The Australian Methylamphetamine Market: the national picture*, a complementary intelligence report released in March 2015, Chris Dawson (the CEO of the ACC) said the 'availability and addictive nature' of crystal meth had 'created new demand in urban, rural, and disadvantaged communities. Stay-at-home, low-income parents with less education, living in country areas indicated notable levels of trying ice and using it compared to other groups.'

Those who are unemployed are more likely to take meth, as are gay men, labourers, and people who live in regional and rural areas. A 2015 Commonwealth Scientific and Industrial Research Organisation (CSIRO) study found that the prevalence of methamphetamine use was likely to be higher in Indigenous than non-Indigenous communities. A 2011 report from the Burnet Institute of Medical Research found that 30 per cent of female meth addicts said that weight loss or maintenance was the primary reason for their first use of the drug. And there is certainly a stage in meth abuse when people consider you at the peak of your attractiveness — this is before the sores develop, and your body shows the signs of malnutrition. I noticed that when I had my quarter-life meth addiction at the age of twenty-seven, people complimented me at first on my weight loss, one person noting I had a 'boyishly thin' figure, and another saying I had lovely cheekbones. It is impossible to sustain this state, however; before long, I began to look like Skeletor with acne.

Many people use meth to help them work. This provides the perfect counter to any suggestion they have a drug problem, or that the drug is detrimental to their life. Because, of course, if you hold down a job and earn money, then, in theory, nobody can criticise what you do to either maintain or unwind in your spare time. The Victorian parliamentary inquiry said that it found 'witnesses presenting to the Committee have spoken of the use of methamphetamine to get through tight deadlines, long hours including double and triple shifts, and just to "get through their working day".'

In an article published in August 2015, Nicole Lee wrote that:

> Most people who use methamphetamine are employed (nearly 70%) … Some industries have a higher level of use than the general population. These include wholesale trade, construction, mining, hospitality and manufacturing, and people in trade, technical and unskilled workers are also more likely to use. Some people start to use methamphetamine to manage workplace conditions, such as long or late night working hours or jobs that require a lot of focus or a lot of confidence.

What I noticed when I was using (and still non-psychotic) is that when I was high on meth, I would do a lot of certain types of work, like moving stuff around and organising files. I would become completely shut off; I could do repetitive work for hours on end without feeling bored—I wouldn't need to eat, drink, sleep, or even go to the toilet.

In essence, meth makes you like a machine—exactly the kind of machine that would fit neatly as a cog in a capitalist economy. In his book *Methland: the death and life of an American small town,* Nick Reding examines the collapse of small town mid-west America in the face of globalisation via the prism of how meth slowly came to grip the region. Noting that meth and amphetamines were born pretty much at the same time as industrialisation, Reding asserts that poor and working-class Americans had been consuming the drug since the 1930s, whether it was marketed as Benzedrine, Methedrine, or Obedrin, for the simple reason that meth made them feel good and allowed them to work hard—a valuable part of the American liberal ethos of 'superseding class through hard work'.

It is worth asking, though, whether meth is genuinely performance enhancing, or whether it is only effort, or even just confidence, enhancing. A drug counsellor told me she once worked in a hotel overlooking a 'gorgeous Sydney beach', where she worked alongside a woman who always came to work on speed. This woman always seemed extremely busy, contented, and productive. One day, when my counsellor sat down on a break with her boss, he whispered to her, 'She [the speedy one] seems to be working hard all the time. But when I actually look at what she has done, she is doing far less than everyone else.'

So does meth improve performance or does it turn people into ratty robots who put in twice as much effort for half the result? While some studies have shown that meth's performance-enhancing features are more perception than reality, there are a number of dissenters to this view: Carl Hart (the Columbia University associate professor we met in Chapter 2) not only thinks that the harms of meth are often exaggerated, but he also suggests that meth can actually *improve* brain function, at least in the short term. His research, he says, shows that:

> Low to moderate doses of amphetamine can improve mood, enhance performance, and delay the need for sleep. But repeated administration of large doses of the drug can severely disrupt sleep and lead to psychological disturbances, including paranoia.

I have noticed that among many meth users there is the sense that when they take crystal meth—as illegal and taboo as it is—they are asserting their freedom and autonomy in a media-saturated world where our minds are constantly at risk of being colonised by marketers, talking heads, trite TV show plot-lines, and terrible newspaper articles. It is a way of feeling in control. And yet, for me, when I was up, I was about as authentic as someone in an advertisement. That said, though, meth can make you feel as if you are fulfilling the goals prescribed by capitalist society. You are left feeling as if you are winning by cheating, and that everyone else is stupid. You feel as though you have unleashed your productivity, and your creativity, and your self-actualising potential. Perhaps this is where the feeling of liberation comes from—the feeling that there is only you, and that what you feel is all that matters. Users get this feeling because meth allows them to think of life as their own personal dream—and in a dream, the dreamer is the only one who is truly alive.

Slovenian philosopher Slavoj Žižek says fantasy is the central stuff of ideology, and that in psychoanalysis, fantasy is a lie that covers up holes in our existence. He says the 'tragedy of our predicament' is that at the very moment when we think we are free, when we escape into our dreams and fantasies, 'it is at that very moment that we are within ideology itself'. Many drug users associate taking drugs with liberation from conventional ways of thinking, and as a way of generating new ideas. This can certainly be true, although crystal meth often makes people's fantasies of themselves and their life-narrative mere reproductions of the societal ideals that they think they are transcending. So while I *did* experience a breakdown of illusions, I went on to form a far more simplistic, self-serving imaginary world. Meth made me self-obsessed, atomised, work-focused, and egomaniacal — traits that many might describe as the defining tenets of our age.

And of course, when the advertisement ended, and the laughter at thinking I was living in such a world had died down, I would be miserable for at least half a week, in stark contrast to that world where all my dreams were coming true. Most of the time, a person's descent from meth-user to meth-addict isn't a dramatic one: at first, it's a series of thoughts or feelings, rather than an abject act of destruction or negligence. The user-come-addict will most likely attribute the cause of these feelings to something other than the drug, and if questioned about their addiction, they will be quick to assure you their use is not problematic: they still work, haven't raped a cat, and haven't mutilated their genitals. When *my* dream bubble burst, I was left lying on the couch with the curtains shut, emotionless and sombre, as if a nuclear holocaust were occurring outdoors. And who wouldn't want to live full-time in a television advertisement when the alternative is a constant feeling that you have the flu, and in which the easiest way to deal with your negative feelings is to take more crystal meth?

## Chapter Ten

# Into the Vortex

A FEW YEARS back, I met a 60-year-old guy named Bernard; he was smoking crystal meth in a public area in a gay sauna. I was between addictions, and so I didn't join in — I just listened.

Bernard was a very skinny, extremely well spoken, former private-school teacher. He was, first and foremost, polite and dignified. He talked in a kind of pure poetry, with just the right amount of detail, poise, and rhythm. He was old-fashioned, genteel; it was almost as if I had met the ghost of Patrick White. As he smoked more meth, though, he began to resemble Mr Burns from *The Simpsons,* specifically the episode in which Mr Burns is found in the woods and mistaken for an alien. His voice became higher-pitched as he told me: 'I had a good job, I was on a very good salary, I had a nice house, and I was very well-respected in the community. Then I met Crystal, and she wrapped her sweet, toxic tentacles around my heart and never let go.'

As the night wore on, he explained to me that when he smoked crystal meth, he could sit for hours on end with his eyes shut, imagining himself climbing mountains and surviving snow avalanches, or going on heroic journeys through deep tropical jungles. 'Once, I sat there for three straight days and explored these caves until I found the ruins of an ancient underground kingdom with huge castles and pyramids. When Crystal ran out of her love, I went and got more so I could continue with the adventure.'

This would often continue for up to eighteen hours at a time. After years of going on these adventures, Bernard woke up to find he no longer had his job, or his salary, or his house—all of which, in turn, led him to smoke more meth.

Jack Nagle was a tall blond basketball-mad 19-year-old living in Melbourne's south-east suburbs when he decided it was time to broaden his horizons.

'I wanted to get out in the world, start mixing with people who weren't from my high school,' he told me. 'I guess there wasn't really anything missing in my life, I just wanted to try new stuff, meet new girls, that kind of thing.'

Along the way, Jack stumbled across crystal meth. Curious—having already dabbled in other amphetamines—he smoked a bit, and then a little bit more, and then the next weekend, and the one after that, and then during the week, until he was lost in a fog of thoughts, ideas, and theories.

At one stage, he went on a 10-day binge, where he smoked more than $7,500 worth of meth and was consumed by fantasies, starting with the recurring belief that he was at the airport waiting to get on a plane to Thailand, when he was, in fact, in his bedroom. He told me that after a while, 'I became convinced it was all part of a TV show plot, and that my life was a TV show, and I was being filmed all the time.'

'Like *The Truman Show*?' I asked.

'Yes,' Jack replied, 'exactly like *The Truman Show*,' and he went on to relate how he had once confronted a girl (who had rejected him) about her role on this TV show—she, quite naturally, freaked out.

'Eventually, I started kind of performing for the camera,' he explained. 'So one day I got home after a day of smoking, believing that the cameras were on me, and I thought to myself what a boring day it had been, and that the viewers probably would have been really annoyed with me. So I stood up in my lounge room and broke out in this mad dance for fifteen minutes just so the audience would be entertained.'

One winter evening in Perth, in 2014, Cassy McDonald took an intravenous shot of crystal meth in her suburban home and, almost immediately afterwards, heard her phone ringing. 'For some reason, I felt really desperate to answer it, like it was some king of emergency,' she said. 'I had this feeling it was my mum calling to tell me something really important.' Having decided that the phone must be somewhere in her car, she went out to the car, which was sitting unlocked in her driveway, and began to search.

'All I remember was fear; I was terrified, I locked all the doors and refused to get out, and ripped open all my dashboard and seats looking for the phone. It seemed like I was only in there a few hours, but I was in there for two whole days. I only came out when my partner's sister pulled up with my son.'

After a long conversation with her sister-in-law, Cassy realised that not only had she been in the car for almost forty-eight hours, but also that she didn't even *own* a mobile phone. Cassy had been experiencing a drug-induced psychosis, and in fact, as a former dealer, she has seen more than her fair share of people having psychotic episodes.

'There was one girl who came over and started plucking out all her eyebrow hairs. At first her eyebrows looked pretty good, but she just couldn't stop. When she had not a single eyebrow hair left, she started on her hairline.'

I put these three stories together to begin to illustrate the link between crystal meth and what we might call, at its simplest, *imagination*. In broad terms, this refers to the ability to form new images and sensations in the mind that are not perceived through the five senses.

What Bernard, Jack, and Cassy describe is neither a daydream, nor mild paranoia — instead, these experiences are all encompassing and self-generating, and produce complicated narratives and/or visions within a state that often blends, and then sometimes confuses, metaphor for reality.

I call this state the Vortex: powerful, self-perpetuating, highly graphic, highly detailed, highly imaginative, rolling-stream images and ideas that flow in your mind whether you like it or not. They can be utilised for creative purposes; alternatively, one can get stuck in the 'movie', or fall into error, thereby taking them literally and entering what modern medicine would describe as a psychotic break.

The Vortex can be an irresistible force, often offering a visual narrative that is far more exciting than the here and now, and sometimes far more exciting than what some users will otherwise do in their entire lives. When I met Bernard, I hadn't experienced the Vortex but I *had* experienced psychosis in the form of delusion.

By contrast, when you're 'up' in the 'Fantasia' of crystal meth you re-imagine yourself, and often your life, in a more favourable light: you become your ego-ideal. This, however, can also lead to a sense of victimhood. As you lose your sense of empathy and perspective, you may also begin to perceive the bad things that have happened to you, or the bad things you have done, as being the fault of other people. You may become egotistical and extroverted, often sharing inflated stories of achievements, as well as stories of how other people harmed you, in an exaggerated and paranoid fashion.

In my experience, the Vortex — at least in the early days of my crystal-meth use and abuse — followed Fantasia; it usually occurred when I was alone. The images and ideas are far more vivid than Fantasia, so vivid that you almost can't do anything other than experience them—they don't just float in the background like they do in Fantasia, and they are often hard to articulate, especially during the experience. The Vortex is a highly individualised and usually compulsive experience; fantasies rage through your head without the slightest bit of effort—but often these fantasies are not about yourself, your fears, or your desires, although they can be. There is often a waking, lucid-dream-like feeling to the Vortex, and not long after moving into Smithy's, I entered this strange new world.

On one of the first nights at Smithy's during which I took crystal meth, I remember he was entertaining three guests in his bedroom, one of whom was Beck. He had music playing loudly, and I could hear them talking over the top of it. The smell of bleach from a hard-core cleaning session was hovering in the air. I had the overhead light off, the lamp on, and I was typing away at old notes from my rehab days, trying to pull together an article. I was typing away effortlessly, rhythmically, quickly, and without judgement. Soon there were 1,000 words on the screen, then 2,000, and then, as two hours passed in a few heartbeats, I had 4,000 words written.

I had a break to make a cup of tea. As I was standing in the kitchen, leaning against the bench, I started seeing very vivid images of people I had once met at Mardi Gras. They were living in an alternate dimension that looked like rural Queensland centuries ago. A few minutes later and I had written up these images as best as I could, but I was struggling to keep up with them as they joined together, becoming more like a movie. As the night passed, I would either be trying to write these images down, though often struggling to articulate the detail, or I would become so enraptured with them that I would just stop and sit on the couch to enjoy the show. People would appear in elaborate, original costumes; the valley and surrounds created themselves, conversations began, and plots thickened.

This was my first experience of the Vortex, and I loved it. When I started to become conscious of what was happening, though, I got into a bit of a panic. I began to see this process as a kind of creative ecstasy that could yield very positive results; but then it seemed that the more I willed it, the more I wanted it, the more I brought my ego into it, the less vivid and self-generating it became.

To return to the night in question, though—at around four in the morning, I became aware that Smithy's guests had left. This occurred to me because Smithy was hovering around me, pinching his crotch. He was hovering like … let's say, a cat that had just swallowed a bird, or a kid about to ask their parents for money.

Smithy had a tendency to mumble when he was on crystal meth, though it was nonetheless clear to me that he, too, was having wildly vivid fantasies of his own. At this early stage of me living in the house, though, he seemed hesitant to give away the detail of his visions; it was almost as if he were giving me bits and pieces of what he was thinking to either get me to fill in the gaps or to get me interested.

Eventually, these hyper-sexed images of his broke into my already dwindling creative stream, and in turn started another self-perpetuating, perhaps even clearer, image stream that I struggled to switch off—a rolling movie of crazy, hot, sex. The Vortex, it seemed, had grown a libido, and the images even had a Fantasia-like quality, featuring me performing as a sexual champion with various lost and unrequited lovers.

After a short time, I moved into my bedroom and started masturbating to this self-generating porn that seemed as if it had been made just for me, with all the people I liked best, performing the most erotic acts I could imagine.

I found these images totally captivating, 'even better than the real thing'. In the 'real thing', people weren't at my beck and call; the actual world, with its limited opportunities, rules, and *actual other human beings* was always going to run a distant second place to a magical alternate reality where I was the star and nearly anything—and everything—was possible.

So there I was under the blanket; the light was off, and I was pulling and pulling, and I didn't want these movies to stop, and I kept pulling, but I couldn't seem to ejaculate. So I kept going, and then I saw, from under the plastic blind in my tiny bedroom with nothing in it but my bed, that it was starting to get light outside.

I remember thinking that it must have been at least an hour that I had been masturbating because it had become day. No matter how hard I tried, though, I couldn't ejaculate. The 'movies' just kept getting better, and I couldn't stop watching them: for one thing, it felt as if I wasn't actually in control of them or of anything I was doing. And, naturally, I was also enjoying being there.

I think it's fairly well recognised that sexual fantasy can express more than just sexual desire, and that the things we fantasise about are not necessarily those we want to do in real life. But I found the sexual fantasies I experienced in the Vortex to be especially morally complicated; they presented me simultaneously as who I wanted to be, and who I would never, ever want to be.

And yet the more unpleasant and unclean the fantasies became, the more exciting they seemed. When I finally finished, I pulled the blanket off myself; my hair and face were as wet as if I'd just got out of the shower, and it seemed as if the daylight had been part of the Vortex: it was clearly still dark outside. So I got up and walked into the kitchen, where Smithy looked at me in surprise.

'Where have you been?' he said.

'What time is it?' I asked.

'It's about 8.45.'

'8.45 at *night*?'

'Yep—where you have been all day?'

'All day?'

'Yep, you were gone for ages,' Smithy said.

'What day is it?'

'It's Sunday night. Have you been in that bedroom all day?' Smithy asked.

Yes, I had. I had been masturbating for sixteen hours non-stop, and it felt as if I had been in there for less than an hour.

Beck was also there, and took me into the bathroom to say, 'Smithy thinks you've ripped him off. He's been going on about it all day. He reckons you didn't give him money for the gear last night.'

'I didn't, Beck, I mean I haven't, I haven't left the house, I've been, well, masturbating all day. For sixteen hours,' I said.

But this information didn't seem to register—Beck was very concerned, but only about Smithy. It seemed that Smithy's imagination had run off on a tangent of its own; he may well have pictured me sneaking out the house, laughing to myself that I had taken his drugs without paying, adding details such as I had been planning it all night, or that it had been revenge for the argument we'd had.

So I sat him down and explained to him that I hadn't left the house all night, and would give him the money after I got back from the main street, where I was going very shortly, and his face lit up in relief. This seemed to pop a dark fantasy of his own—started, perhaps, when I had left him alone while he was talking about sex, thus triggering his sore point.

Here let me make the following point about fantasy—Smithy's fantasies that he knew were fantasies, and my fantasies, which I also recognised as such, also seem to be the basis of psychotic thinking. While it was rare that I myself would be experiencing the Vortex as real, it does seem to me that the Vortex may reveal a nexus between creativity and madness. It is perfectly possible that these trains of thought—psychosis, imagination, fantasy, and creativity—exist in one inter-connected line. But in some cases, for reasons that might be related to genetics or trauma or underlying neurosis or depression or meth dosage, people take these fantasies to be actual reality.

Twenty years ago, Rebecca McKetin did a PhD on whether repeated amphetamine use could cause psychosis in lab rats. At the time, this was considered a fringe topic in Australia. Today, McKetin is an internationally renowned expert on the links between crystal-meth use and psychotic meltdowns. In her long-term study, introduced in Chapter 2, McKetin found that methamphetamine users are five times more likely to show symptoms of psychosis than non-users. The study also showed that the greater the dose, the greater the risk of psychosis. The risk of psychosis also increased with the severity of dependence, and dependent methamphetamine users were a particularly high-risk group for psychosis even after adjusting for a history of schizophrenia and other psychotic disorders. The study also found that other factors often associated with regular meth use, such as lack of sleep, a history of trauma, and the concurrent use of alcohol and cannabis, also increased the odds of psychosis.

While the link between crystal-meth use and psychosis is firmly established, the link between creativity and psychosis in the context of crystal-meth use has never been empirically studied. Dr Glenys Dore, the clinical director and a consultant psychiatrist at the Northern Sydney Drug & Alcohol Service, and a clinical senior lecturer at the University of Sydney, told me that the problem with establishing that link is that researchers would need to connect an MRI machine to someone while they were using crystal meth and performing a creative task—an ethical and funding quagmire.

Dore, a friendly, vivacious woman with a kindly tone and slight Kiwi twang, went on to say, 'But certainly we know that crystal meth works on the limbic system of the brain, which is also partly responsible for creativity and imagination. Also, what I think some of these experiences tell us is that not everyone has a terrible experience with the drug, and that some people do find the drug very useful in having new, creative experiences.'

Crystal meth increases dopamine in the brain, the same hormone the brain is flush with when we orgasm. High dopamine levels are not only associated with anxiety, schizophrenia, and aggression but also with compulsive behaviours, sexual addictions, *and* creativity.

Making connections between things that are otherwise considered disparate is characteristic not only of psychosis, but also authentic creativity and new scientific discovery. One of the most remarkable thinkers alive today is a woman named Nancy C. Andreasen. Dr Andreasen is the Andrew H. Woods Chair of Psychiatry at the University of Iowa's Carver College of Medicine, as well as the director of the Neuroimaging Research Centre and the Mental Health Clinical Research Centre there. She is a prominent neuroscientist and psychiatrist, but her first career was as a literary scholar, and she was a professor of Renaissance literature at the University of Iowa for five years. She has written many books, and created many original theories on the science of creativity.

Andreasen says her research shows many things: that creative ability has no correlation with IQ; that creative people are more likely to have immediate family members with schizophrenia; and that creative insight is more likely to happen when the mind is relaxed. She has interviewed many high-functioning, highly creative people, and also taken imaging of their brains while they complete a creative task. She says creativity is about 'coming up with a lot of ideas very quickly' and is essentially a process called 'divergent thinking', which she defines as the ability to come up with a large number of responses to an open-ended probe; this is in contrast to 'convergent thinking', which tends to apply a sequential series of steps to answer a question that has only one possible solution.

Andreasen has noted that many (not all) of the highly creative people she has studied describe being in a dreamlike state when they produce creative work, and that these 'unconscious processes' are important for creativity. She gives the historical example of Coleridge, who once 'composed an entire 300-line poem about Kubla Khan while in an opiate-induced, dreamlike state, and began writing it down when he awoke; he said he then lost most of it when he got interrupted and called away on an errand—thus the finished poem was only about a quarter of the size'.

While it is, of course, possible to reach these creative states and produce creative work without using crystal meth, in retrospect I feel that my use of crystal meth helped illuminate some of the key ingredients in producing creative work—to let myself be a kid again, that kid who was playing in the backyard and creating an entire world around him. Moreover, I had to let go of my rational mind, surrendering control and giving precedence to an apparently more rudimentary, silly, imaginative part of the psyche that often serves no rational adult purpose.

After that first weekend in the Vortex at Smithy's, I was determined to make the most of these self-generating images. I thought the best way to handle this was to use in low doses, sit myself down at a computer as soon as I had a dose, and concentrate on putting energy into creative ideas.

Poetry, songs, more ideas for novels followed. Songs? Yes—while my dad is a musician, and I used to sing as a young teenager, I have never played an instrument, played in a band, or done anything remotely musical as an adult. Yet here I was, writing and performing songs—even if they weren't exactly worth listening to.

What happened next is evidence of my increasingly delusional state. One of the reasons I began writing music was that I had met some professional musicians when I was in Sydney who were exceptionally kind and who had invited me to a few events. During a conversation with one of them—a well-known performer from London—at an after-party, he told me that I had a made a 'boring choice' to become a lawyer when I obviously enjoyed doing creative things, and he asked me if I ever felt like writing music.

When I was high on crystal meth, I would daydream about these events, and eventually decided that these musicians had deliberately sought me out because they believed me to be an extraordinary talent who could be a professional musician, and that they had started me on something called 'The Journey'. I even believed that, at times, the performer from London was sending me lyrics for songs via telepathy.

At other times, these delusions would darken, and I believed that they had invited me to the events in order to *pretend* that they wanted me to become a professional musician, so I would make a fool of myself on stage, and they would get revenge on me for a long list of other nasty things I had, in turn, done to other people throughout my life.

Smithy, meanwhile, seemed to experience his fantasies (which were usually sexual in nature) almost as an entry into another world. There seemed to be some kind of twilight zone, in which he started to experience his visions not as happening there and then, but as a *memory* of something that had happened—and not a scene that he had directly seen, but instead one that was hidden from him. These fantasies often involved Beck, and blended with his terrible sense of persecution and rejection.

For instance, one night, about two months into my living at

the house, Smithy was standing in his bedroom. He was in typical form, hovering around the mirror with his face covered in ever-growing pus-y sores and a serious look, as if he were pursuing something immensely important in life, all the while wearing an undersized campy T-shirt (mine) with his guts pouring out the bottom.

This was also a night when one of those sores had become infected and inflamed. When he finally turned around, one particularly rabid concoction underneath his eye had become a huge abscess, about four centimetres square.

In much the same way he treated his face, when Smithy talked, he kept going back to the same thing over and over again — infecting and inflaming and making it worse. His fixation on this evening was a particular something that either did or did not happen on New Year's Eve at his mum's holiday house. Although he wasn't in a relationship with Beck at the time, he had invited her, along with some friends, to spend a few days at the house over the New Year period. He had become convinced that something had happened between Beck and one of his friends — something that Beck denied, and that was further confused by the fact that they had all taken acid and meth.

At times he was sure I was somehow in on it, and that I was hiding information from him. The truth was simply that I found Beck's denial more convincing than his paranoia, and I believed that his paranoia had its origins in a waking fantasy he had willed himself to experience.

It's hard to say what flicks the switch between fantasy that you know is fantasy and fantasy that somehow feels as if it's real. The ecstatic creative impulses I had initially experienced became harder and harder to control and come by. Most of the time, in fact, I would stop coming up with creative ideas, and just masturbate for ten to fifteen hours, enraptured by my own sexual fantasy world, or I would engage in grandiose fantasy about the praise I would get for a finished creative product, rather than actually doing the work. This represented a downgrade from the Vortex to the self-centred world of Fantasia and inevitably, when the drug was wearing off, I would focus on how other people had jeopardised my creativity; how my parents, being so focused on class, had stunted the creative areas of my brain; and how being a full-time creative was my destiny.

I would still experiences patches of the Vortex among all this, and would usually disappear into the garage to write songs and poetry, and jot down ideas, though I did find it tiring. In between the worlds of Fantasia and the Vortex, highly unusual thoughts would come bursting into my head. I spent many an afternoon battling against psychotic thoughts. I would tell myself, 'No, you have had meth today, and this is *not* the time to try to work out ambiguities or mysteries or things you have been unsure about; you are bound to make a wrong turn.' So many things didn't make sense when I was in these states, and I couldn't handle any kind of grey area—I needed absolute answers.

Psychosis makes lots of different things, sometimes everything, feel as if it is connected in very sinister ways; there is no real beginning, end, or in-between. That said, when I describe my psychosis, it's hard to capture what it is actually like—if you are someone who has gone through a psychotic episode, then you will know that reason and language are often completely transformed: time loses meaning, and your recollection of events is littered with mysterious blackouts—so that ideas which took six hours to form, or behaviours which took a whole day to build to, can seem as if they all happened in an instant when you reminisce, or try to explain what happened to someone who wasn't there. The blackouts also mean that it's very difficult to determine when you started to make a strange turn in your logic. Sometimes I had ideas that happened in a flash, or built up over a day. At other times, I would come in and out of psychotic ideas over different meth trips, and they would build steadily or change shape over the course of several weeks.

I know now that psychosis was just my imagination at work: a combination of higher-functioning abstract ideas and a literalist, infantile, regressive imagination creating a straight train of thought that broke down the border between metaphor and reality, subject and object, self and other, inside and outside, then and now. When you're in psychosis, doubt falls out the window: there are often very few uncertainties, and you feel as though you possess all the facts. By proxy, you can believe you know what everyone else is thinking, and that they must know what you are thinking, too. This is why people who are having psychotic episodes often talk nonsense: you know what you mean to say, but you talk in complicated metaphors about this secret/special thing because you think it's what everybody is talking about, even when they sound as though they are talking about something totally irrelevant. When you finally piece things together in your psychotic logic, the world stops seeming so chaotic; everything just kind of slows down, and the world assumes a perfect shape with sharp ends and a clear, if unsettling, order. There are secrets being uncovered, epiphanies being had, and metaphors being interpreted.

One day I started having invasive thoughts about things people had said on Facebook that I didn't understand. The more I thought about these references, the more it seemed like everyone, collectively, was making fun of me. At the time I was also freelance writing, so I thought I would go over to Beck's and check the computer to see if my article had been published. I googled my name, and some key words from the article, and nothing came up — instead, one of the first hits to come up was a blog written by an American musician of the same name. When I clicked on this blog, which was showcasing this other Luke Williams' new music, it struck me how poorly written and self-absorbed it was.

I immediately thought that everyone was making fun of me and had invented this satirical blog to send me up.

Because I found it so incredibly clichéd and poorly expressed, I decided that it must be a parody. A parody of me! And, for some reason, I linked this back to my failed attempt at doing a show at triple j — that somehow the people behind this were people who I used to work with at the station, who were making fun of me. And when I went back to my Facebook feed, it looked like all my triple j ex-colleagues were making coded allusions to me, and how lame I was, in their status updates. I contacted a trusted friend, who was able to talk me down from my delusion, and soothe me, at least momentarily.

Dr Michael Eigen, in his book *The Psychotic Core*, describes the experience of the psychotic individual as one of opposing extremes: 'At times, it seems that the psychotic person dissolves their mind in order to rebuild themselves. Or he may seem to search grimly through its debris, leaving nothing out, as if he were looking for something essential, but still unknown … The flux itself becomes fixed and imprisons him.'

And yet, for me, the psychosis would often just fall apart very quickly, and I would feel clearer and more enlightened than usual. The paranoid delusion would just become too big to sustain itself, there would be too many people involved in it, and I would realise how wrong I had been.

One night, when Smithy kept going on about Beck and New Year's Eve, I asked him why he was so worried about it — given that *if* it had happened, it had happened when they weren't even together.

'Concentrate on yourself,' I said, and he looked at me with a glimmer of surprise. 'What would you like to be doing with your time? I mean, I know you're a full-time dad, but what else would you like to do?'

'Play cricket,' Smithy whispered like a little kid.

'So why don't you start playing again?'

He didn't respond.

'I reckon you don't want to play because you like to be good at everything, and you're scared that if you start playing again at your age, you won't be any good at it. I understand that, Smithy. I reckon we're actually quite similar.'

And upon hearing that, he nodded, staring into the distance, and said, 'I love cricket, I miss it, I miss it,' and started to cry. I got him some tissues, waited for him to stop — which took no more than a few minutes — and then I said, 'Let's talk about something else.' It was like a neurosis was smashed open, shattered, and then evaporated that night; Smithy never talked about New Year's Eve to me again.

## Chapter Eleven

# Parents and thieves

I WAS STANDING inside an indoor shopping centre in a middle-ring suburb, with the smell of potato cakes, and kebabs, and Kentucky Fried Chicken not so much lingering but dominating the air amid the cheap clothing stores, the buzz of a hundred voices murmuring at once.

I was with two young crystal-meth users, Samuel and Jodie. Both were in their early twenties: Samuel was bone-thin with blue eyes and very white skin, and his wife was a heavyset Italian. They were not every-day-of-the-week, skin-falling-off-their-face addicts, but they *did* pay for their habit with crime. And, just to clarify, they didn't start committing crimes when they started doing meth. Samuel, then twenty-two, had been doing so-called petty crimes for almost a decade.

I had come along to see how they generated cash through crime. For a few weeks prior, I had seen them coming back to Smithy's from their crime sprees with hundreds of dollars — all obtained by stealing from department stores, and not by visiting pawn stores, which are a sure way for the amateur criminal to get caught.

Samuel had a slouch when he walked; he wore a cap and

fluorescent worker's clothes to make it look as if he'd just come from work when he walked into a store. Much of his behaviour was subterfuge, designed to detract from the fact that he had sticky fingers and a smooth, deceptive tongue. He was disarmingly slight, and one could easily interpret his accent as that of a good, hard-working man: a furniture removalist, a labourer, or a factory worker.

Samuel had been in jail, and he knew the kind of crime he was carrying out is considered petty and not worth the risk — more manipulative than masculine. It didn't involve violence or weapons or gangs, and yet he still took pride in telling me that his trick would earn 'six hundred bucks in less than hour … it might be petty, but it brings in the cash and I have never been caught'.

And on that note, he asked, 'Are you ready?'

'Yep,' I said, wanting to play it cool, and not show how excited and nervous I was. We walked through the entrance of a low-end department store; Jodie came in behind us with their 18-month-old son Greg in a stroller. Both said hello to the female bag-checker, who smiled approvingly at them and their baby.

'Come with me,' Samuel said, and he took me down the aisle. 'Now find the smallest, most expensive thing you can, and put it in your pocket.'

'What about security bleepers?' I said, too loudly.

'Keep your fucking voice down. Those bleepers are an illusion; there's nothing on most of this stuff that actually causes them to go off. And nobody is watching those cameras. It's all a fucking illusion, nobody is watching, I've been doing this for years.'

On one level, perhaps, Samuel was worth listening to. Or, at least, he was an authority on this particular subject. He hadn't worked for a long time. He didn't care what other people thought. He had developed an apparently ingenious technique for avoiding all the responsibilities that plague so many of us. He had cheated the system, beating alarm clocks and irate bosses—and meth was part of his 'perfected' lifestyle. In a world where choice is apparently so prevalent, but finding a genuine counter-culture is rare, Samuel used meth and crime to live a lifestyle that he considered superior to everyday human experience.

Indeed, there is a definitive link between meth and crime. People who already commit crime often take meth because it fits with their lifestyle. This may skew the statistics: this cohort would probably commit crime whether they were taking meth or not. Other people use meth to give them the Dutch courage to commit crime. And as for manufacturers of meth, it is not uncommon for them to coordinate sophisticated robberies of amphetamines and amphetamine precursors from pharmacies, chemists, and pharmaceutical warehouses.

A two-month research project into police detainees in key areas around the nation conducted in 2015 by the Australian Institute of Criminology found that 61 per cent of those held at Kings Cross police station in Sydney tested positive for amphetamine, as did 40 per cent of those who ended up in the Brisbane City watch house, and 43 per cent of those in East Perth.

Results from a New South Wales Bureau of Crime Statistics research study revealed that heavy users of amphetamine—those who reported at least sixteen days of use in the month prior to arrest—had 53 per cent more property offence charges (like stealing or trespass) recorded at arrest compared to detainees who were less frequent users and non-users. Higher rates of property offences among methamphetamine users were also associated with younger individuals, being unemployed, and having reported illicit use of benzodiazepines in the thirty days prior to arrest. According to the Australian Institute of Criminology, between 1999 and 2012, 20,402 police detainees tested positive for methamphetamine. The highest proportion of charges recorded against these detainees were property offences

(26 per cent), followed by violence offences (24 per cent).

Detective Leading Senior Constable Jason Bray told the Victorian parliamentary committee that one of the biggest problems police face with meth-related crimes is that career criminals who use it are able to be much more active:

> When people are taking this drug, they are able to stay awake for three, four days on end … In the last year, for instance, we had a career criminal that I have known for probably ten years. In the past he may go out and do a burglary or a break-in of some sort, once every week or two weeks, depending on what his circumstances are at the time. On this particular night he did upwards of 20 crimes.

The inquiry also heard from the Victorian Aboriginal Legal Service, who reported that, based on reports from their solicitors and client service officers, ice was making their clients more likely to offend, either to 'fund their habit' or 'because ice makes them more likely to take risks'. In 2013, South Australian District Court Chief Judge Geoffrey Muecke told the *Adelaide Advertiser* that methamphetamine-related cases were 'clogging up' the court system. 'In a normal arraignment list of say 30 cases, there will be I think at least half ... either trafficking meth or supplying or manufacturing, or there are assaults and/or robberies to feed an addiction,' he said. 'It's probably the most highly addictive drug that we've ever had.'

It must have been halfway through my time in the house when I met another, um, 'interesting' character at Smithy's house. His name was Jake; he was twenty-seven, and had grown up in southern New South Wales. He took me outside to smoke cigarettes with him while he ranted about how Australia was no longer Australia, about how there were no longer enough houses or jobs for Australians because there were too many immigrants coming in, and about how said immigrants were taking over, and fuck the kind of society we were living in, and so on. I never even pretended to agree with him, telling him instead that it sounded rather like 1990s Hanson-ism to me, as well as slightly fascist. It wasn't until the next time I was at the library using a computer that I realised how entrenched his ideas were. I had a Facebook friend request from him, and his profile pic was of an eagle with a swastika. A few weeks later, Jake came over with his girlfriend, who I noticed was looking teary as she stared at the television. I asked what was wrong, and she didn't hesitate to tell me that they were living at her sister's house in Cranbourne because they couldn't get a rental house, Jake couldn't find a job, and she was too scared to apply for a housing-commission house because she was worried that Human Services would be notified, and they would take away her kids because of their crowded living conditions.

'Everybody thinks I am a bad mother,' she told me. 'But I'm trying my best … every rental I apply for has over a dozen applicants and we don't even get a look in, and I think it's because Jake has a criminal record.' I offered to help in any way I could, including writing letters and organising for her to see a social worker, while quietly thinking to myself how appalling it was that there would no available housing in a low-budget suburb surrounded by hundreds of kilometres of cleared, sparsely populated farmland that, for reasons I could not understand, was *not* being used to build low-cost housing.

His girlfriend never came back, but Jake would come over and smoke crystal meth now and then. To his credit, and for all his anger and problems, he never got hooked. Every time he came over, he thanked me for hearing out his girlfriend, and would always offer me cigarettes, or some of his meth. Politics were not discussed, but one day, when I had my back to him as I was watching television, he was talking about how great he was in bed and I replied, 'I find that very hard to believe; if you had confidence in your own ability to fuck, perhaps you'd stop feeling the need to be such a fascist fuck.' He cracked up laughing and proceeded to tell me, in great detail, how he could make a girl orgasm.

As I turned around to look at him, I saw that, unbeknown to me, the daughter of one of Smithy's clients had been standing at the door listening. I don't know how old she was, but she was standing there in a school dress; once Jake finished his lengthy description, he turned and stared at her.

About a month later, on a Saturday night (or perhaps I should say Sunday morning—it must have been at least 1.00am) I had given Smithy some cash, which I knew he had spent on drugs with Jake. But on this night, he hadn't given me the dose, and I was very much in the mood for it. Instead of my drugs, I saw Jake standing in the front doorway dressed in a navy-blue hoodie, and black tracksuit pants covered in dried plaster.

'Where are you going?' I asked, which was really code for 'where is my meth?'

'Just off to work, honey,' Jake replied.

'Work? What do you mean work? You told me you haven't had a job in years.'

'Work—I'm going to work,' he said again.

'What are you talking about, work—I don't understand.'

'Now Luke, let me get this straight,' Jake said. 'You've studied law, you used to work as a journalist at the ABC, you have two degrees ...'

'Yes,' I said.

'And you can't work out what I'm doing?'

'Um, no,' I replied. 'That's why I'm asking.'

'Has anyone ever told you that you're a dumb fucker with a good CV?'

'Just tell me where you're going.'

'To find you some common sense,' he said.

And he left, and soon thereafter I sank down a couple of bongs, struggled to get a word of sense out of Smithy—who was, as he was so often, preoccupied with his face in the mirror—and promptly went to sleep.

When I got up the next morning, there were three brand-new fridges and a new washing machine in the kitchen and dining area.

'Jesus, what's with all this new stuff?' I asked.

'You really are a dumb fuck,' Jake replied.


There is among all this a far more difficult reality to digest—the presence of kids.

When Cassy McDonald was in her early twenties and dealing drugs—all day, every day—she had one trio of regular customers who would offer to clean her house in exchange for drugs.

'A grandmother, a mother, and a daughter,' she told me. 'Gran was about sixty, the mum was thirty-nine, and the daughter was eighteen. I would give them a point of meth between them, and they'd clean my house from top to bottom, cut my lawn, and then go over it with nail clippers to ensure the blades were even, wash and iron all my clothes, even stuff that was brand new.'

Cassy's mother also used meth—as Cassy found out when she started using herself at the age of seventeen. 'It all added up,' she told me. 'My mum has always had big mood swings—she always had people over, and she never slept.'

Intergenerational meth use is more common that you might think. Geoff Munro from the Australian Drug Foundation told me that it's relatively widespread, often involves grandparents, and is 'deeply problematic'. Dianne Barker from St Luke's Anglicare in Bendigo told the Victorian parliamentary inquiry that she had been involved in a case where a mother was facilitating the delivery of ice to her children while they were in residential care in St Luke's.

In other cases, the children of meth users don't live long enough to share in the lifestyle. There are stories from all around the world of people and parents who slip over the edge and fall so deep into the pit they can no longer see the cliff from where they fell. These stories never cease to horrify. There is the 25-year-old Californian woman Jessica Adams, who after a 4-day meth bender returned home from a party ready to crash. And crash she did, with her 2-month-old son asleep next to her. At some stage during the night, she rolled over in her sleep, suffocating the baby to death. Across the border in Nevada, meth addict Bransen Locks was charged with shaking his girlfriend's 1-year-old to death while on a bender. An autopsy would reveal the baby had 'midline shift' of the brain after the incident. In Wales, former Lostprophets frontman Ian Watkins said he was on crystal meth when he engaged in an online sex session via Skype in which he instructed a woman as she sexually abused her infant for his entertainment. He later sent another woman a message saying he wanted a 'summer of filthy child porn' and spoke of a desire to 'cross the line'. In the Slovak Republic, a 4-month-old baby was left brain-dead after his parents gave him crystal meth to stop him crying. In Phoenix, Arizona, the 5-year-old daughter of a meth user tested HIV-positive, after the girl complained about her mother sticking her with needles in late 2014.

Research published in the *Child Abuse & Neglect* journal reported that kids said their parents would become 'aggravated', 'angry', and fight a lot, and one third of children who had parents who used meth reported that their parents became violent. Other children complained about not getting meals or not being taken to school. Throw in paranoia, depression, and the three-day-long sleep marathons after a binge and things are bound to go wrong. While I certainly saw evidence of this in the way Beck treated her daughters, what I found more difficult to discern was the kind of parent Beck might have been if she didn't take meth — it seems possible, given her self-centred reasons for having children, that she would have pretty much behaved that way anyway.

Dr Keith Humphreys, professor of psychiatry and behavioural sciences at Stanford University, describes crystal meth as a 'seductive' and 'powerful' drug that affects the part of the brain that signals our most essential functions including safety, eating, sleeping, and taking care of children. It is his view that the drug 'takes over' and leads users to believe that meth can replace these essential functions — hence why, in many cases, kids are neglected by their meth-using parents: the drug is competing for 'resources, attention, and love' that would otherwise be given to them. Dr Humphreys claims he has made contact with child-protective services over the issue, and says that some children are being sexually abused by their meth-using parents — a consequence, he says, of meth destroying both empathy and sexual inhibitions.

Academic Susan McFarlaine, who has researched families living with amphetamine problems, writes that amphetamine-using parents may become 'withdrawn, self-focused, paranoid delusional' and are likely to be preoccupied with 'planning, obtaining, and using drugs as well as emotionally and physically affected by ATS use and the subsequent withdrawal and craving'.

From my own experience, the effect of meth use on parenting is far more subtle and far harder to detect than outright abuse. I saw parents slowly lose interest in their children, their instincts apparently lost in the fantastical fog of regular use. One user I interviewed, Mark McNeil, told me he used to live for his daughter, and for his family, but they soon became not so much second-rate as utterly irrelevant in the face of his addiction. In typical meth-addict style though, even after his wife divorced him, and there was a court order preventing him from seeing his children, he didn't believe that he had a problem.

And how were Beck and Smithy's children faring in this culture? Beck's oldest daughter Hayley, who was now fifteen, seemed to bear the brunt of Beck's bad temper. If Beck wasn't screaming and yelling or threatening violence, she was crying. Hayley spent more than half of her week staying at a friend's house. Whenever I came over to stay, Beck and Hayley would have a terrible fight, and I would spend an hour talking it over with Hayley in her room, where she would sob and tell me how much she disliked her mother.

'She's worse when nobody is home, and it's just us kids,' Hayley said.

I am not sure why I never said anything to Beck—I guess I wanted to be the peacemaker and I was usually glad it wasn't directed at me. I wish now that I had said something: it was Hayley who gave me my first taste of unconditional love as an adult. When Hayley was a toddler, she cried when I left the house. I spent hours with her, talking to my feet after I drew faces on the soles of them, turning them into a cheery old-fashioned married couple called 'Sally' and 'Bob'. Sometimes I wondered if the only reason I stayed with Beck was because of Hayley; I always felt that the more people she had involved in her upbringing, the better. Beck's yelling and screaming was always worse on Christmas Day—as if to pre-empt and quash any suggestion that she should have gone without pot that week, and spent a bit more on gifts. I always tried to supplement Alice and Hayley's Christmas with gifts; one year, when I bought Hayley an expensive camera for Christmas, Beck asked me why I nor anybody else bought *her* presents.

Hayley was highly intelligent; she won awards at school, won premierships at sport, she was attractive and well-dressed, and was always in the popular gang at school—all of which was quite inexplicable for those who knew the circumstances in which she was raised.

Many of those who played a part in Hayley's upbringing—and there were quite a few of us who did—want to take credit for Hayley. The truth is, though, that she was just born with something special about her.

She was like a mysterious otherworldly plant who sucked up the shit around her and turned it into beautiful flowers that attracted anyone and everyone. She was independent, and preferred her peer group to home life, although that was hardly surprising.

About three months before I moved into Smithy's, I was staying at Beck's on a visit from Sydney. On the walk back from the doctor's one morning, Beck happened to drive past me (she had spent the night at Smithy's). She stopped the car on the side of the street, crying hysterically. When I asked what was wrong, she said she had a cold, and when I rolled my eyes, having heard it so many times before, she told me Smithy had done something to her. I was in no mood for her drama, and just kept walking. I ended up at Smithy's for the afternoon, and when I didn't return at night, Beck called, still crying, demanding to know why I was spending my time with him and not her. So I went back to her house, where she told me again she had sinus pain, and ran to her room to cry for an hour.

That night, Hayley came back and asked to talk to me in her room.

'Mum is a bully ... she screams at me all the time, over nothing, she calls me names—I just can't live here anymore.'

(By this stage, Beck and Smithy had split up. He had a restraining order against her, and Beck—despite her best efforts to contain it—was starting to crumble.)

When I left that time around to go back to Sydney, I sent Beck a long and thoughtful Facebook message telling her that I was worried about her behaviour and that I thought the way she was behaving around her kids may have been damaging. She never replied, and later admitted to me that she'd never read the message.

A few days after Christmas in 2014, Hayley — still fifteen — contacted me to say Beck had kicked her out of the house on Christmas Eve. Apparently, the camera I'd bought for Hayley a few years earlier was missing as well, along with several other things from the house, and Hayley told me that — along with some of her niece's things — Beck had sold them in a pawn shop.

'I know I'm not sixteen yet, but I really want to move out,' Hayley said.

She explained that there was a family who were happy to have her move in. She gave me the mum's number and I rang and had a chat with her — the family were church going, liberal-minded, and reasonably well off. The mum told me that the kids had set dinner and homework times, and that they loved Hayley to bits. They were happy to have Hayley stay as long as she wanted, and would look after her like she was one of their own.

I agreed to support Hayley in moving out and to help organise her Centrelink, and told her not to tell her Mum that I had helped her. Beck was deeply hurt when her oldest left the nest at such a young age, and I think she would have wiped me from her life if she had known that I'd helped her move out.

So while I'm really not sure what sort of parent Beck would have been if she had not been a drug user, I do know that crystal meth's ability to dull everything else so you keep feeding on it undoubtedly made her less of a parent that she might have been. The way meth works on the brain probably explains the relatively high number of women who continue taking meth while pregnant. In 2013, at the Royal Women's Hospital alone, 15 babies were born to mums who had used ice during their pregnancy.

Their paediatrician, Dr Ellen Bowman, told me that some of these babies are born showing withdrawal symptoms, meaning they could be floppy and refuse to eat, and be undersized or irritable. She said the long-term risk with these babies could be that they grow to be adults with undersized heads. Research by journalist Kate Legge, in an article published in *The Weekend Australian* magazine, also found that pregnant mothers using ice was a growing problem, with numbers increasing at those hospitals that screen mothers for substance abuse (which many do not).

There are also many examples of minors getting involved in meth irrespective of their parents' actions. In their submission to the Victorian parliamentary inquiry, Melbourne City Mission report that workers in their early-intervention programs have identified meth use in 'clients as young as 12 years of age' and that '70 per cent of [their clients] between the ages of 14 and 15 years of age have had some experience or use of ice'. The Victorian component of the 2011 Australian School Students Alcohol and Drugs (ASSAD) survey found that approximately 5 per cent of 17-year-old male and female secondary school students had previously used amphetamine for non-medical purposes at least once in their lifetime. The same survey showed 1 per cent of high school students aged between twelve and fifteen have used amphetamine or methamphetamine in the last month.

Suzi Morris, community services manager for Lives Lived Well, the super-clinic formed after the merger of the Alcohol and Drug Foundation Queensland, the Gold Coast Drug Council, and the Queensland Drug and Alcohol Council, told *The Courier Mail* that young adults and teenagers using drugs was becoming more common.

'I would say 15 to 24 is a common age group. There are a lot of street kids and a lot of kids who have been traumatised. They don't have loving and caring homes, they are couch surfing and they are vulnerable.'

More generally, if there are lots of teenagers using crystal meth, there are lots of very worried parents. Or, at least, I hope they are worried—and worried in a reasonable, proportionate, rather than hysterical, way.

I know, for instance, that I gave my parents more than a few headaches when I was staying in Smithy's house. During our conversation on the night my mum talked me out of the idea that she and everyone else were poisoning me, I made the link between my psychosis and what I had been through in high school. A painful exchange between Mum and me followed:

'I know what this is all about,' I said. 'Do you remember why I had to leave high school?'

She hesitated as if she were struggling to remember.

'C'mon, Mum.'

'Because you were gay?'

'Yes. Did you know there were people at my school who believed gay people should be killed?'

Silence.

'Well, Mum, there were, and that's why you shouldn't be surprised that I have delusions of people wanting to kill me.'

And on and on I went.

'And how come none of you noticed what was going on? It felt like you were in on it at times.'

She stayed silent, and I guess—in retrospect—listened attentively as I detailed the awful things that went on in that high school, things that I have outlined in this book but am usually reluctant to talk about. She remarked on how horrible this must have been for me, but the more I talked the more I *wanted* to talk, and the angrier I became. Mum kept on bringing the issue back to drug use, a move I regarded as superficial, and which made me even angrier again.

The conversation spanned many hours and I shed many tears; at times, I regressed to adolescence, and said many of the things I wished I'd been able to say when I was that age.

A few days after that conversation, my mother rang me and

said 'You have to come home, Luke, you have to get away from the drugs, you have to come home right now!' with many tears and much drama. It was beginning to remind me of high school, when she'd kicked me out of home. No doubt she was bitterly disappointed by my choice to start using crystal meth. My parents had paid $8,000 for my graduate certificate in law, and had then given me more money to go and live in Sydney.

Although we still fought fiercely, as my drug use increased I was ringing her at least once a week during a psychotic episode — she was actually very good at bringing me back to earth — and eventually she stopped pushing me into coming back home.

One of the reasons she probably got off my case was that she could tell that in between meth doses — I was usually close to being back to normal then — that I was trying to fill a gap in the twins', now aged five, lives. The boys lived at Smithy's, at Smithy's insistence. He wanted to have full custody of the boys as he claimed that he didn't trust Beck with them because of her 'foul temper'. After Beck's crack-up at Smithy a few years earlier, their break-up, and the subsequent restraining order, his mum had helped pay for a solicitor to ensure he got custody of the boys.

Beck was largely absent from the house, and although Smithy was a decent dad, the drugs meant the twins were often placed in front of the television for hours at a time. I had noticed that they weren't getting much individual attention, or any of the extras that went with that. I bought them reading books, and textas, and blank paper. One twin liked to sit with me at my computer, pretending we were doing work for our 'boss'. The other liked colouring in and creative games. That same twin was well behind his brother in his reading and writing, and, no matter how much time I spent with him, he was unable to pick it up. The thing that I found most troubling about both boys was their speech, which was particularly poorly developed: a combination, probably, of twin-talk, being raised on cartoons, and not having been enrolled in kindergarten, though they were well overdue.

At her worst, when I tried to talk to Beck about the twins, she'd sit there with a sour expression on her face, barely looking away from the TV screen, occasionally rolling her eyes as if I were simply showing off. When I told her about the learning difficulties of one of the twins, she commented only that he must have 'Smithy's slowness', because the other twin didn't have the same difficulties.

As I was not using very much for the first six weeks, I was also getting the twins' breakfast for them — after a few days on the gear, Smithy would go into these micro-sleeps from which nobody could wake him. So the twins would come into my room at about 10 o'clock in the morning:

'Weet-Bix, Uncle Luke,' one would say. 'Get out of bed *nooowww*,' the other would yell before they ran off laughing. After I poured them bowls of cereal, one would usually say, 'Thanks, Uncle Luke, you are the bestest uncle in the whole world'. Not quite — there were times when I saw them, played with them, and looked after them when I was on meth, and while I don't think they were directly harmed by this, I can now see that the risk to them was high, and I believe it affected the sanctity of our relationship.

I had fallen in love with the boys long ago, but now I felt a sense of responsibility for them; I was genuinely worried about their fate if I left the house.

The department store was still buzzing along with the smell of potato cakes and the nonsensical chatter. I was waiting in line with Samuel, who had managed to stuff no less than six printer cartridges in his pants and under his top. These printer cartridges were worth $53 each. Samuel was making a purchase — a packet of Smith's salt and vinegar chips — both to make him look less suspicious, and to get him a branded plastic bag, which was crucial for the next stage of his operation.

After charming the cashier, Samuel paid for his chips and—just as he had predicted—walked through the security gates with over $300 worth of stolen goods.

He texted Jodie, who followed him through the same checkout a few minutes later. Her purchase was chocolate; when we got back to the car a few minutes later, she revealed more secret compartments in the baby's pram than you'd find in a military bunker. These compartments were filled with DVDs and CDs—perhaps about $400 worth.

'Now we go to the next store,' Samuel said.

He drove us twenty minutes down the road to the next suburban shopping mall, which had the same department store. He walked up to the customer-service counter with the six printer cartridges in the bag with the department store logo, where he was greeted by a young and rather flirtatious clerk, who listened attentively as Samuel told her he'd just realised he'd bought the wrong thing.

'As it turns out, you don't sell the cartridges I need,' he said. 'My ex-wife is really angry with me—we need the printer for a big school assignment, and I've spent all my cash. Can I get a refund?'

The clerk scanned them and said, 'Well, I can see they're from here. I can give you a refund, but I will need to record your ID.'

Samuel handed over his fake ID, and the clerk entered some data, and then handed over $318 cash.

'Oh, thanks so much,' he said. 'You're a life-saver,' and the girl glowed with satisfaction.

Samuel didn't celebrate until we were a hundred metres or so away from the store.

'Now what?' I asked.

'Time to get some meth,' he said. 'Want to join?'

'Why not?' I replied. 'Why not.'

## Chapter Twelve

# The devil

WHEN FORENSIC PATHOLOGIST Dr Isabella Brouwer examined the corpse of 18-year-old Ultimo woman Jazmin-Jean Ajbschitz for the coroner, she noted that the injuries were consistent with and typical of the kind of blunt-force trauma injuries she saw in catastrophic car accidents.

Specifically, she noted that the force of the impact that killed the teenager had crushed the right side of her ribs so badly that her heart had almost been torn in half. Dr Brouwer's examination also revealed bruising on Jazmin-Jean's left shoulder, her left leg, right arm, lower back, upper back, her scalp and the left side of her neck, multiple rib fractures, and haemorrhaging to her tongue.

All fairly standard car accident injuries, right?

As we learned in Chapter 1, though, the hard-partying 18-year-old with olive skin and a kindly manner was brutally killed by Sean Lee King, her long-term boyfriend, in her own apartment.

The pair had originally met at a music festival, and things were good between them for the first three months. But over time, Jazmin-Jean found him jealous and controlling. He would read her text messages to and from other people, and demanded to know where she was at all times. Drugs became part of the mix, and in the few months before the murder they had been arguing about meth — Jazmin-Jean was worried they were both using too much of it.

On the day he killed her, Sean Lee had been smoking crystal meth, and had drunk an entire bottle of bourbon. The pair argued throughout the afternoon, mostly via text message, before she seemed to dump him in a text in which she also called him a 'cheating, girl-bashing dog'. He called her back, and Jazmin-Jean and a female friend who was with her put him on loudspeaker where they heard him say, 'I'm going to fucking kill you. Wait until I see you. You don't know what I can do.'

Sean Lee made his way to his now ex-girlfriend's unit block on Harris Street, Ultimo, on the city fringe. He began yelling at her from outside, in the black of night, amid the high-rises, the terrace houses, and the semi-new public-housing blocks. Jazmin-Jean eventually came outside, hugged him, and invited him inside.

Twenty minutes later, she was dead.

When police arrived at the scene, they found bloodstains on various parts of the hallway that led to the bathroom, as well as on Jazmin-Jean's scarf and one of her shoes. They saw blood smeared on an adjoining wall, and more blood staining the floor of the bathroom. Faecal material had been deposited in the shower recess — it is thought that Jazmin-Jean was so terrified in the last moments of her life that she lost bowel function.

Sean Lee was arrested and faced trial. The 27-year-old told the court that he'd only killed her because he was high on crystal meth; he said that he didn't intend to do it, and didn't remember doing so. And it is true both that Sean had never killed before, and that meth has a reputation for being a deadly drug, an evil drug — a drug that is known to have been involved in many homicides and violent crimes. Indeed, few dispute that there is at least *some* link between methamphetamine use and violent behaviour.

McKetin's 2014 research, as quoted earlier, found that people become more violent when they use more ice, and this propensity increased if the person experienced psychotic symptoms. The researchers found a six-fold increase in violent behaviour when chronic users take the drug: while only 10 per cent of users were violent when they were *not* taking the drug, this increased to 60 per cent when they were taking crystal meth in heavy doses. In the United States, a 2006 study from Ira Sommers and Arielle Baskin-Sommers from the School of Criminal Justice and Criminalistics at California State University interviewed 205 meth users in Los Angeles, and found that 26 per cent of them committed violence while under the influence. Further to this, although a slim majority of those had committed violent acts when they were *not* on meth, 46 per cent of the study participants who committed violence reported that they had never committed a violent crime prior to the methamphetamine-based events. The researchers concluded that for those individuals 'chronic methamphetamine intoxication produced a paranoid state, including frightening delusions that often resulted in aggressive acts. The nature of these acts overwhelmingly took the form of intimate partner violence.'

Based on experience, I have to agree that if you take enough meth over a long enough period of time, it can open one's own heart of darkness, until one's system is flushed with the darkest bloodlust one may ever know. What is bloodlust? In this context, it is a feeling of excitement about committing a violent act—as if all your life had led up to this moment, and your cruellest, most playfully sadistic behaviour will be your legacy, your act of revenge: a most dramatic and symbolic way to be remembered.

You may remember Rebecca McKetin's explanation that meth users are effectively 'paranoid from too much dopamine, irritable from low serotonin, and overhyped—all at once'. And for some users, this biochemical reaction plays out in shatteringly real ways.

Nicole Millar—an attractive mother of three with dark-brown hair and bright-blue eyes—had fought off her own share of drug and alcohol issues over the years. But in June 2010, at age forty-two, her life was relatively stable; after spending half a decade working as a cleaner, she now worked as a driver for an automotive spare parts retailer. She drove the youngest of her children—Kane—to school every morning, kept herself busy at her job, where she was well liked, and spent most of her nights relaxing with her kids at her public-housing house in Bayswater—a fairly rough but reasonably pretty town shadowed by the hills of the Dandenong Ranges in outer south-east Melbourne. Nicole was known as a quietly spoken woman, and a naturally gifted caregiver, but there was one problem she hadn't yet been unable to free herself from—attracting highly abusive men. Nicole had already fled a violent relationship in 2005, an event that led into her public housing. In 2008, she began seeing 37-year-old David Hopkins, a nightshift tunnel-worker/foreman at the local Eastlink freeway, which was then still under construction. The pair felt immediate chemistry, and it wasn't long before David moved in. Nicole would soon find out that David—a tall willowy man with olive skin and light-brown hair—had a foul temper and propensity for drug use.

By 2009, things had turned sour, and Nicole asked David to move out. He did move out, but trouble continued as the relationship continued in an 'on again/off again' state: on 19 November 2009, 15-year-old Kane Read was at home when Hopkins burst into their family home. He smashed up a wardrobe and a mirror in Nicole's bedroom. In May of 2010, Kane and Ashlea, Nicole's daughter, noticed Nicole had marks on her arms, a bruised eye, and a cut between her eyebrows. She initially said that she received the injuries from tripping over, and she refused to blame Hopkins for it, though he would later admit the injuries had occurred when he threw a book at her under the influence of magic mushrooms. Despite this, they did have periods of getting along apparently quite well, and they still spent time together.

On the first day of winter 2010, Nicole was in the car with David as she drove Kane to school. Hopkins had taken testosterone and had been drinking alcohol the night before. He had also been smoking both hash and crystal meth. The pair then drove to a Safeway service station. Kane later testified that when he'd observed them talking ten minutes earlier, they had been getting along just fine.

At 8:16am, as David was filling the car with petrol, he took the petrol pump nozzle out of the petrol tank and carried it to Nicole's door; at the same time, he pulled a knife from the left side of his belt. He then re-entered the car through the passenger door with the nozzle in his right hand and the knife in his left—he aimed the nozzle at Nicole, and began pumping fuel all over her. She was screaming for help and continuously sounding the car horn. David responded by pointing the knife at Nicole, and stabbing or slashing her in the neck and throat area while continuing to pour petrol over her. Nicole had a strong instinct for survival, and she tried frantically to get out of the vehicle; Hopkins—pumped on meth and steroids—overpowered her, dragging her back inside the car. He took a cigarette lighter from his pocket, and lit the petrol on Nicole. Covered in fuel, Nicole immediately caught on fire from head to toe. She stumbled out the driver door engulfed in flames.

For a period of precisely three minutes and twenty-one seconds, Nicole sat on the forecourt of the garage, burning from head to toe. Horrified witnesses attempted to get to her to extinguish the flames. One person had a fire extinguisher. But all who came towards her were threatened by David, who was still holding the knife. While preventing them from coming to Nicole's aid, Hopkins also verbally abused her as she sat in agony.

Nicole fought hard for her life. Police arrived on the scene and arrested David. Nicole was flown by air ambulance to the Alfred Hospital, where she arrived at 9.45 in the morning. She was still conscious, writhing in pain. The doctors assessed her injuries as being non-survivable. An anaesthetist attended her at 10.00am, putting a tube in her throat, and administering an anaesthetic so that she would fall into a deep sleep. Just before she lost consciousness, a barely recognisable Nicole—whose milky-white skin was a melting mess of red and black burns that had covered 90 per cent of her body—told the anaesthetist, 'Please don't let me die'. However, the staff already knew there was nothing they could do, and at 6.00 that night, she died in her sleep.

It's the fate of Nicole Millar, and others, that led many to call meth what it seems to be: an evil drug that makes ordinary people commit horrendous acts.

On 27 March 2014, the *Herald Sun* published an article that reported that ice had been linked to the killings of fourteen people across fourteen months in Victoria.

Mr Clive Alsop, a Magistrate at the Latrobe Valley Magistrates' Court, told the Victorian parliamentary inquiry that he had observed a direct link between ice and domestic violence: 'In one region of Gippsland a major resource has been set aside for the assistance of women who have to leave home because of domestic violence [and] 100 per cent of the people who are seeking services at this person's establishment are there because of ice-related difficulties.'

And Dr Andrew Crellin, director of Emergency at Ballarat Health Services, told the inquiry that one of the main problems medical staff faced when dealing with meth users was their high levels of aggression.

Given how horrific meth-related crimes can be, and how often they occur with apparently little or no motive, it is not surprising that we commonly hear that meth not only leads to evil acts, but is itself an evil drug. Amid this genuine and legitimate outrage, though, is a complicated question of accountability — to what extent can we hold a person legally and morally responsible for an act they carry out when they're using meth? Is it the drug or the person? And if it's a combination of the two, where exactly do we draw the line between them?

In my own experience, I believe that there are a number of factors contributing to the way I behave when I'm on meth. I have a family history of psychosis and a personal history of trauma. I have a tendency to engage in reckless behaviour and an even higher tendency to develop addictions. I have also identified that while I had persecution fantasies when I was younger, and still did when I was older, once I started using meth, these were replaced with grandiose fantasies of inflicting needless pain on others. Which I can only put down to the fact that I had, at various times in the preceding years, taken testosterone to increase my muscle mass, as well as doing heavy weightlifting and kickboxing classes. I believe this changed me, both physically and psychologically. As I will explain further in this chapter, testosterone figures in many meth-related murder cases — both Sean Lee King and David Hopkins had a long history of using anabolic steroids in the lead up to their brutal acts.

Another thing that these murders have in common is that in each case the perpetrator killed his partner. Men killing their wives and girlfriends is a social issue that is discussed far less often that it should be. And methamphetamine, at least until very recently, has received far more media attention than domestic violence, though I imagine the impact of the latter is almost certainly both more common and more devastating. Domestic violence is the leading cause of death and injury in women under 45 in Australia, with more than one woman murdered by her current or former partner every week. And yet, it is often the case that when these murders are reported in the media, they are done so in the context of methamphetamine rather than the longer-standing, wider-spread problem of male violence against women. Is it easier to blame an 'evil drug' than to address issues of patriarchy, or to peer into the 'evils' occurring in the western institution of the family?

Now seems a good time to introduce Beck's younger sister Stacey, and take you to the day, in the summer of late 2009, that changed her life. It was a warmish evening, and the then 26-year-old had just arrived at her Pakenham home. She had come from a day at TAFE, where she was studying early childhood education. Stacey had a distinct sense of satisfaction after she ended a day at TAFE: she was the first of her sisters—the same sisters who loved to torment her about her weight, her lack of hygiene, and her lack of luck with men—to study at a tertiary level.

Sometimes when Stacey (whose weight has fluctuated between moderately overweight to morbidly obese throughout much of her life) would get home after a hot day, sweaty and bothered, one of her sisters would yell out 'the fat bitch is home'. Often she was too tired to fight back, but when she did, it was a sight to behold. I once saw her hit Beck in the head with a broom. So I guess when her sisters threw those verbal attacks they knew it was bear-baiting and they knew awful consequences might follow, but they did it for the thrill.

A few years after Stacey left high school, she still hadn't had a serious relationship; she had been having casual sex, though, and she fell pregnant with twins in her early twenties. At this time, like many other times, Beck's ex-partner Nick was back in jail, and he would occasionally ring Stacey for a bit of a chat. Stacey would be happy enough to keep him company, and was even happier the day he told her that he had a friend in jail who had seen photos of her and was keen to meet her.

He was an older guy who liked big women, Nick explained, and he thought Stacey was very attractive. Stacey was at first sceptical, not because he was in jail — she knew many men who had been to jail, men who were flawed but essentially decent — but because, in her experience, she'd found that guys who claimed to like 'bigger girls' were often simply looking for an 'easy root', or someone they could degrade during sex. When Stacey first spoke with the man on the phone, she found him to be self-deprecating, broken, and genuine: a 'nice guy'. She had daydreamed about having a criminal boyfriend like her sister — she thought it was glamorous and exciting, and he made her feel sexy and wanted. He said things to her that no man had before, and soon she was making plans for them to meet when he got out in three months.

Naturally, Stacey interrogated the man — Mick was his name — about why he was serving such a long sentence. He explained that as a young man in a rough, tough Queensland town in the late 1980s, he'd become caught up in drugs and with the wrong crowd: a bikie gang who paid him to do seemingly innocuous jobs. One day, Mick recounted, with more than a tinge of sadness and regret in his voice, his boss had explained that a man owned the gang money, and it was his job to do the 'deed'. Not on his own, of course, but Mick was told if he did not assist a couple of heavies in killing the debtor, he would be digging two graves: one for the debtor and one for himself. So Mick reluctantly, and in a haze of alcohol, pot, and speed, had helped in the murder of a lower-chain drug dealer who owed tens of thousands of dollars, and assisted in disposing of the body. He said thinking of his actions now made him feel sick to the stomach; that he still had nightmares about it; that he was a changed person.

He told Stacey she was absolutely beautiful, and within a few weeks of his release, and after more than eight years in jail, Mick met up with a heavily pregnant Stacey.

The couple would wed, have another baby together, and have — apart from Mick's casual meth use — a fairly normal, non-eventful, crime-free, working-class life. They both worked, they were debt-free, and had been together for nearly eight years on the day Stacey arrived at their modest but respectable three-bedroom brick home in Pakenham, tired but upbeat. She had overcome no shortage of nastiness and setbacks to get to where she was: a home, a husband, three kids, an education and a good job, stability, and good friends.

Cleanliness was still not her strong point, though, and as she walked into her messy lounge room, a waft of unclean dishes in the air, she saw Mick's legs sticking out from the end of the couch.

He was supposed to be at work at his factory forklift job, a half-hour's drive away, in ten minutes.

'Bloody get up,' she said, trying to hold back her laughter.

'Oh shit, I must have dozed off,' he replied, and the skinny little man with brown hair, blue eyes, tattoos, and a 'tail' got up, rubbing his eyes, and hurried out the door saying, 'I'll only be a little bit late'.

Oddly enough, he took her car not his.

'He must have been half-asleep,' she chuckled to herself.

When she peered out the front to call the kids in later that evening, she noticed that the numberplates were missing from Mick's car.

'That's weird,' she thought. 'Typical bloody Pakenham,' assuming that someone had stolen them from the car while it sat in the driveway; at the time, petrol prices were very high, and she thought they were most likely to have been stolen by a petrol runner.

She rang Mick, who expressed surprise and agreed that he would need to go the police tomorrow to report it. He arrived home that night while she was asleep, and the next day he seemed particularly annoyed about the numberplates going missing. He said he was worried, given his criminal record, about driving the car without the plates and being caught by police. Stacey needed to take the children to a maternal-health service fifteen minutes' drive away—she agreed it would make more sense if she, rather than him, drove the un-plated car.

As she sat in the waiting room, flicking through some magazines, her mobile rang.

'Hello, is this Stacey Hughes?'

'Yes.'

'This is Sergeant Brady from Pakenham Police.'

'Okay.'

'We have just intercepted your husband Michael.'

'Right?'

'We've pulled him over because we believe he has assaulted a female. He has, in turn, informed us that he has a crystal-meth addiction. He has further informed us that you have his Commodore. We're not concerned that you are driving it without number plates, but we need you to bring this vehicle to Pakenham police station for the purposes of evidence.'

'Um, yes, okay—but can I ask what's going on?'

'We think that Michael might have been trying to harm himself because of depression related to his crystal-meth addiction. Before you bring the car down, I need you to tell us if there is a black satchel in the car.'

After Stacey went to check the car, and confirmed the satchel was there, the officer asked her to check for a rope, which she also found.

Stacey cancelled the appointment with the maternal-health nurse, and drove back through the winding roads of Cockatoo and through the bushy back roads of upper Pakenham.

Her thinking was incoherent and rife with uncertainty and

contradiction. She knew he had been using meth: she'd found used syringes around the house, and she knew he disappeared into the garage to use. For the most part, though, he had been easier to get along with when he was using, and he'd also get a lot done around the house. Stacey couldn't help wondering if this whole situation could have been avoided if only she had stepped in and said something about his meth use, rather than just enjoying the apparent side benefits of it.

She handed the car over to the police, and, a short time later, Mick came out of the cop shop and got into Stacey's car. Mick was physically smaller than Stacey. She was a woman who had often fought off her sister's vicious verbal attacks with brooms, fists, and a ferocious anger that would leave many a grown man shaking in their boots.

He started talking once they began driving. He told her he felt terrible about what had happened, that he knew he had fucked up, and that he needed drugs counselling. Stacey just stared ahead as Mick talked about how his meth use had gotten out of control without him realising, and how he'd been so depressed on the 'day in question' that he'd driven himself to Emerald Lake, intending to hang himself in the bush.

Emerald Lake is a plain, muddy lake, surrounded by natural waterways and a rather stunning jumble of native and introduced species, with the largest nursery in the southern hemisphere—the Puffing Billy tracks run right through it—separating what is rickety Australian bushland from what looks almost like medieval European forest.

It was at this junction, where the native bush meets the introduced forest, that Mick said he was preparing to hang himself. He was just preparing the noose when, in a state of meth-psychosis, he saw what he thought was the devil coming towards him. Petrified, thinking perhaps he had somehow 'already crossed over into hell', he grabbed the devil and wrestled it to the ground.

Moments later, he realised it wasn't the devil—it was a jogger with a red hoodie on who was actually trying to save his life. He ran off, bewildered, and yet somehow shocked to his senses; he got back into his car and drove off.

Still Stacey didn't answer, though her bemusement had turned to curiosity. She knew Mick had been through some terrible things in his life, and his meth use had been at least daily for quite some time. As the car pulled into their driveway, Mick said he wanted to keep talking for a little while in the car. He lowered his voice and rested his head in his hand.

'It was just my way of escaping,' he said. 'I've been through so much awful stuff with my family, and what I went through in jail.'

She let him back in the house. Although she was ambivalent about his story, she was worried that he didn't have anywhere else to go, as well as the fact that if his story were true, then homelessness would be an extraordinarily harsh price for him to pay. The next day she took him to the doctor, where he repeated what he'd told her the day before, pledged to get off the meth, and got a prescription for anti-depressants and Valium.

On the day of the court case, some five months later, Stacey sat in the pews at Dandenong Magistrates' Court. They had been waiting all day for the committal hearing to begin. She had decided to put aside her suspicions and her prejudices, and deal with what seemed to her to be the facts. The rope, which suggested he had tried to hang himself, and his meth abuse, which suggested he was having psychological problems, and his mostly very good behaviour since he'd gotten out of jail.

They entered the courtroom just after 3.30pm. She sat behind Mick and his defence team. The case would begin with the prosecution pulling out a huge manila file of evidence against Mick—most of it, to Stacey's surprise and horror, based on his prior convictions.

Even Mick's solicitor was unaware of the vast majority of these prior offences; he didn't have a copy of the file, and his client hadn't told him about most of them. Out of fairness to the defence, the committal hearing was reset, so Mick's solicitor would have time to read the file.

Mick would be free to go, for now, and on the way home he explained to Stacey that most of the offences occurred during the time he'd spent in prison, and were related to drugs, gangs, and weapons—all of which had been to help him survive the tough prison environment.

The next day, sitting in the messy old-school offices of his country-town solicitors, Mick's lawyer said to the couple, 'We need to talk about your criminal history.'

'My history, why?' replied Mick.

'Well, Michael, it might look bad that you were convicted for rape in 1994,' the solicitor said.

Stacey felt herself shut down. He had, of course, told her that he was in jail for murder—had that really even happened?

The clutter in her mind meant she stopped hearing what was being said in that meeting, though she noticed that, by this stage, Mick looked as if he wanted to grow a shell and crawl into it. Stacey knew the ball was in her court. When they got into the car, she deliberately displayed no emotion, instead leaving him to 'fear the worst' as she put on a kind of psychotic calm to keep him on the back foot.

As she drove off, she waited another sixty seconds and then, in a quiet voice, said:

'So Mick, do you want to explain what the fuck is going on?'

'I can't talk about it honey, I just can't. It's not true. There is a truth in it—but it wasn't me. It's a horrible situation, and it's too traumatic to talk about.'

And silence fell upon the vehicle for the rest of the trip.

A week later, and Stacey would find out she was two months

pregnant with his child—their second and her fourth.

A month later, and the court case for the 'devil hallucination' attack would go to court. Mick pleaded guilty, though his lawyers argued furiously that the incident was the result of meth psychosis.

The prosecution's case, however, offered a different interpretation of events. They argued that Mick had acted with cunning and malice: he had snuck up on the 32-year-old female jogger, and he had punched her in the face and thrown her to the ground. This account was corroborated by two eyewitnesses—witnesses that Mick had also seen at the time.

And the rope, the Crown argued, was not even tied in a noose—there was no evidence that Mick was trying to hang himself. There was no evidence, for instance, showing that he prepared himself, a tree, or a rope in any way to end his own life. Following the incident, Mick actually tore off his number plates and threw them in the bushes.

The victim's impact statement stated that she was now suffering daily headaches from the incident, and had moved interstate to escape the intrusive memories.

Mick was sentenced to twelve months.

Stacey was devastated. She knew her sisters would be quietly laughing about it behind her back; she was hormonal from her pregnancy, and largely financially dependent on a man who had been a good provider. Soon she would have four kids to look after, and her mother was only happy to help with her rent as long as Mick was in jail—without him around supporting the family, she worried she would end up homeless.

Despite the evidence and despite her instincts, Stacey decided she would try to accept Mick's version of events. She believed that what he really needed help with was his drug addiction; she wanted to do the right thing for her family, and she wanted to make sure she was treating the cause, not the after-effect. She was deeply conflicted, though, and refused to let him move back in.

At the same time, though, she wasn't quite ready for a divorce. She still wasn't sure how much Mick was responsible for his crime, and how much it was associated with his crystal-meth use — but she was not willing to take the risk of finding out with her children. Mick moved into a boarding house in Dandenong, and not long after he was released from prison, Stacey would receive another phone call to say that her husband had been apprehended a second time, this time for savagely raping a St Kilda prostitute at knife point. Mick denied the woman's version of events, but ultimately it was her word that the court believed, and the last most of the extended family and Stacey's family heard about it was a news story reporting that Mick had been jailed for nine and a half years.

Although Mick claimed meth was involved in the rape, there was no evidence that Mick was using meth at the time, or at any stage in the lead up to the attack. Any suggestion he was acting because of meth or as a result of meth-induced psychosis was rejected by the court.

So, it would seem that meth's reputation can be used by the particularly unscrupulous to attempt to evade responsibility for their crimes. Similarly, it runs the risk of being used by communities to stop them facing up to the more fundamental truths about our long-standing flaws, foibles, and evils.

Let me explain this further: broadly, I see three ways that a person may use methamphetamine as a way to evade personal responsibility for committing a violent act. First, a person may plead 'not guilty' to murder because they were affected by the drug. Second, a person may plan a violent act — and then take the drug — and later use this as an excuse to reduce their charge to manslaughter. And third, a person may lie and say they were on methamphetamine when they committed a violent act, when they actually weren't. A murderer is often not apprehended at the time of the murder, so blood testing for drugs would not always happen. Given that many people think of meth as a transformative 'devil's drug' that makes good people bad, the risks of it being used to evade responsibility in both a moral and legal sense, as well as a way of explaining violent acts to loved ones, remains a significant issue.

So while the panic about crystal meth is understandable, rape, violence, and murder are arguably part of the human condition or, at least, of our society. Demonising the drug allows us to fall back on simplistic, lazy thinking—we run the risk of blaming 'technology' for what is and has always been a human problem. On the other hand, many researchers in the field believe that many murders wouldn't have taken place if it were not for the fact that the perpetrators had taken the drug. In the domestic-violence cases, meth combines with a range of other factors, as we have previously discussed: anabolic steroid use, alcohol, the perpetrator's pre-existing mental-health problems. It makes it very difficult to ascertain what the proportionate response to the drug should be.

Along with the murders of Nicole Millar and Jazmin-Jean, I looked at eight other cases where one person killed another person while on methamphetamine. I picked these cases at random from an Australian legal-database search. I wanted to see what the circumstances were of these murders, how much of a role meth played, and how the court decided on the convicted person's culpability for the act.

Among the eight (10 including Nicole Millar and Jazmin-Jean), I found that none of the perpetrators had committed murder before, but nearly all had prior convictions for violent acts. In four of the cases, the killer (including the killers of Millar and Jazmin-Jean) had been using testosterone as well as meth in the lead up to the murder. In some cases, the killer had no apparent reason to kill the victim, but they did have a complex relationship with the victim. Take for instance, 33-year-old Damien Peters, who in 2001 said he killed his former flatmates and lovers, Andre Akai, 50, and Bevan Frost, 57, after contracting HIV from Mr Akai, and 'suffering years of mental and physical torture'. While Peters' case was the first 'murder-meth' story to make the news—largely because Peters had no history of violence and because he disembowelled his victims and then flushed their organs down the toilet—Peters was actually using a cocktail of drugs, including methadone, testosterone, anti-depressants, and Valium as well as crystal meth at the time of the murders. Peters was sentenced to seventeen years in prison, and the fact that he was withdrawing from methamphetamine and displayed symptoms of 'battered wife syndrome' reduced his sentence. However, it is significant that almost all of the other murders were committed by men who had past histories of violence, including kidnapping and assault. In virtually all these cases, meth was considered to be the factor that pushed them over the edge. In one case, 25-year-old Ross Kondaris killed his grandparents after using crystal meth and becoming psychotic; after examination by three psychiatrists, the court found that he had pre-existing schizophrenia, and could not be held responsible for his crime. He was put on an indefinite custodial order in a psychiatric hospital. Indeed, in this latter case—one of many that Victoria Police had jointly announced as '32 murders associated with crystal meth'—crystal meth was actually *not* considered to a factor in the murder because Kondaris's psychosis was held to be the result of schizophrenia rather than drug use.

Questions of fact and responsibility will ultimately be decided on a case-by-case basis in the courts, depending on the evidence and the circumstances surrounding the criminal act. The diversity of circumstances makes creating a strict rule about meth and personal responsibility seemingly impossible.

At trial, meth use can be argued as either a mitigating or

aggravating factor when a person is found guilty. So for instance, the fact that a person has no prior criminal record and came from an abusive home would often mitigate the severity of the sentence. Whereas a person pleading not guilty, and having behaved in a particularly malicious way toward the victim, would be considered aggravating factors that would increase the sentence length. Drugs and alcohol are traditionally put into the category of mitigating circumstances, particularly if it can be shown that during the act the person was either not fully aware of the consequences of their actions, acted on impulse, acted because of psychotic delusion, or had in some way performed an act that the evidence showed they would almost certainly not perform were it not for the drugs and/or alcohol in their system.

But the courts have (in my opinion very cleverly and appropriately) turned meth's reputation on its head and used it to increase, not reduce, the accountability of people who commit violent acts while high on meth. So if somebody knew *before* taking meth that the drug had a tendency to make them more violent, then the fact the person was on meth at the time of murder will increase the sentence not reduce it. The application of this approach played out in the sentencing of Nicole Millar's killer, David Hopkins.

In sentencing him to a 30-year minimum term, Justice Betty King, an outspoken and flamboyant judge — known for her bright-red curved reading glasses and her inclination to take on some of Melbourne's worst figures — told Hopkins:

> I have viewed the CCTV footage of this horrific event. For a period of three minutes and 21 seconds Ms Millar sits on the forecourt of the garage burning from head to toe … Not only have you doused her in petrol and set her on fire, you then take even more horrific action, in that you then prevented any person coming to her assistance or aid … The behaviour is an

example of the worst kind of viciousness and sadistic behaviour this court is ever likely to see ... Whilst there may be other cases that may also fall into the worst case scenario and possibly even be worse than this it defies my capacity to imagine them. What you did to this woman on this day was unspeakable.

Exactly how much crystal meth drew this highly unstable man into violence is unclear, but Justice King regarded it as a significant contributing factor:

I am satisfied that you were not psychotic either on that day of the murder or for the whole of the previous week, be that a drug induced psychosis or otherwise, but I do accept that you were in a drug fuelled rage ... Rage—drug fuelled or otherwise—is not an excuse, it is no more than part of an explanation for your behaviour. Like the consumption of alcohol and other drugs, it may go some way towards explaining your behaviour which was inexplicable behaviour towards another human being for whom you supposedly had affection.

In the New South Wales Supreme Court in the early months of 2013, Sean Lee King's case turned on his defence team's argument 'that as a consequence of smoking crystal methamphetamine ("ice") and consuming alcohol during the day on which he murdered the deceased, he was not capable of forming any relevant intention' to kill his ex-girlfriend. The defence team utilised a statement from John Andrew Farrar, a forensic pharmacologist, 'that the ability of the accused to form an intention to kill the deceased would have been substantially impaired'.

However, Justice Geoff Bellow, after careful consideration, said that while he accepted that ice increases aggression, and he was satisfied that King was affected by the drug, the fact that King had called 000 after the murder showed he was functioning well enough to realise that his actions would result in murder, and that he had been intending to kill his ex-girlfriend when he started to attack her. And in a ruling consistent with Justice Betty King's approach eighteen months earlier, Justice Bellow ruled that because Sean Lee King knew that ice made him aggressive that 'the offender's intoxication should be regarded as an aggravating factor. It is one which carries with it significant moral culpability for the predictable consequences of the choice that he made to continue taking drugs in the knowledge of their likely effect upon him.'

At this time, it's worth revisiting the conclusions of Ira Sommers and Arielle Baskin-Sommers, who in noting the number of people who became violent while using crystal meth, asserted that developmental factors are also important contributors to violence:

> It has been theorized that the best predictor of future violence is a past history of violence. Accordingly, abnormal deviant behaviour in childhood has been found to be a fairly reliable predictor of aggressive behaviour in adulthood. Much of the evidence that links methamphetamine use with violence is based on clinical reports. Unfortunately, clinical reports are replete with methodological problems. They are limited most severely by their inability to control for the non-drug state or trait characteristics of study patients.

Whether or not crystal meth is in fact the 'Devil Drug'—a drug that may both bring out our worst and also produce a new level of human evil—is still very much open for discussion. One should be wary of anything, however, that resembles a definitive conclusion about human evil, our concept of hell, and the world's most powerful stimulant.

## Chapter Thirteen

# Winter

IT WAS WINTERTIME in the Valley. The cold had closed in, and seemed to be trapped in that flat landscape, which extended to an ocean whose breeze originates in Antarctica and lingers along the Valley's hills.

Smithy would often light a fire in the backyard on winter mornings, and his guests—normally two or three of them, and almost always from the local boarding house—would stand around it in thick winter jackets, looking serious and grim.

If Beck was over, she would be inside, and she, too, would hover, often moving about the house aimlessly: sometimes making a set of curtains on the sewing machine, at other times moving stuff from one side of the house to the other, or reorganising drawers—all with little quantifiable result at the end. Her face was usually pale and wrinkled, and she often had scabs on her chin.

Sometimes she'd bring over spare packets of anti-depressants (we took the same ones), and Ventolin, and food. The food was especially welcome, because at that stage, Smithy hadn't left the house for two months, and wasn't doing any grocery shopping for the boys.

Sometimes she yelled at me, sometimes I had to push her out the door, sometimes she was banned from Smithy's for a couple of days. She would often be having a go at either one of us, but never both at once—sometimes she would listen to us from outside, when we didn't know she was there, and then attack us for saying things she didn't like. Three or four days later, though, she'd return, and it would never be mentioned again.

Always unpredictable, Beck's inner life was, at least from the outside, both a space in which wildly original ideas developed, and a conduit for other people's tastes and desires—by which I mean that she eventually felt these latter as her own. When I asked her about Smithy masturbating in front of me, she assured me that 'he doesn't like you especially, he does this to everyone'.

Indeed, Smithy was often sexually obsessed with whoever was around him, and at that time this included—and was mainly—me. When Smithy would masturbate in front of me and ask for details of my sexual fantasies, Beck would rearrange the drawers, or find some other task that kept her in the room, despite how ill at ease she appeared to be. Her look of bewilderment would gradually give way to a frown, a creased forehead, and slumped shoulders. Smithy, in turn, would miss the subtext—(that she kind of wanted to join in, but didn't; probably wanted to tell him to stop, but couldn't)—and look at her with deep, wondrous suspicion before concluding, and then asserting: 'Stop stealing my fucking pot.'

There we were: taking drugs, living in our imaginations, living out our dreams and nightmares, becoming possessed. My ex-boyfriend Nathaniel haunted me in the years we broke up, whether I was on drugs or not. But on crystal meth I talked about him constantly, I thought about him constantly, I wondered what he might be like now that he was older—twenty-one—I wrote poems about him, songs about him, grieved the mistakes I made, wondered how it might have turned out if we had met a little later.

One day, when I'd had a dose of crystal meth the night before, and was walking around the kitchen thinking about Nathaniel, a visitor to the house said to me, 'I've been keeping track and you've been walking around that bench for seven hours.'

Two nights later, when I was yet again high, our other roommate walked in the door with his young girlfriend. The more I looked at her, the more I thought about it, the more I believed she looked like Nathaniel—short in stature, slightly androgynous, brown hair, brown eyes, dark skin.

Later that night, I started thinking this apparent 'fact' through again, and it occurred to me that at around the same time Smithy and I had had that fight (the one that ended with him on top of me on the lounge room floor of their old Pakenham house) Nathaniel had also broken up with me. I concluded that they had orchestrated this event, because Smithy didn't like the way I treated Nathaniel, and he wanted to turn Nathaniel into a transsexual, so that he and his mates could have their way with the new female Nathaniel. Then, over time, I further concluded that Nathaniel was now named Kristie, and had started a relationship with a guy in that group of friends, who also happened to be Smithy's roommate.

So a few nights later, I still believed this, though I'd also had periods where I believed it to be a delusion, and longer periods where I completely forgot about it. But on this night, as soon as Kristie walked in the door, I looked her up and down, thinking that Nathaniel had done a pretty good job at becoming a woman, except for his shoes, and so I walked up to her and said, 'Everything looks okay, but I don't like your shoes.'

Then I called my Mum again, who once again talked me down, and then sent me a stack of emails telling me that I needed to get off ice and that it was destroying my brain. In return, I told her that she needed to apologise for kicking me out of home, as well as for ignoring the bullying I was going through in high school When she refused, I refused to stop taking the drug. And on it went.

One thing that didn't really change, though, was my belief that I was on The Journey—that some kind of creative discovery was in store for me, and that I was getting closer to realising it.

Smithy would usually ask me if I wanted meth when he was going to score. When I was trying to keep down my doses, and sometimes even succeeding, I would say 'no, thank you', but would often, much to his annoyance and long after the meth had arrived, change my mind, and ask if I could have some. The following happened on one of those nights.

'You bloody always do this, Luke,' Smithy said. 'If you want some, you need to ask me in advance.'

I apologised, saying I would pay him back, and he agreed to give it to me.

'There's only one issue,' he said. 'There are no fresh needles; you're going to have to get a used one out of The Bag.'

'The Bag' was a large, sturdy bag that sat at the top of Smithy's wardrobe. It was a suitably dreadful jumble of freshly used, hepatitis-inducing needles, bloodied swabs, and bent spoons. For future reference, if you ever see a bent spoon with white stains on it, stay away; it is not something you should be using for your Petit Miam.

I kept reaching my hand in and then pulling it out again, as if I had dropped my wedding ring in a bag full of mousetraps. I finally took the plunge, and laid my hand on one of the 50 or so needles in the bag. It had a red cover on it, just like every single other one, and was surrounded by bloodied cotton swabs, and, for some reason, it seemed like the one to choose—who knows, it might have even been mine.

So I carefully picked it out and unscrewed the lid; when I looked down the shaft, I could see a glob of dried blood in the end—it looked like something not even a mosquito would eat, and I almost vomited. Nevertheless, I went in the kitchen and started washing out the needle. No matter how hard I squeezed, and how much bleach I put in the bottom of the syringe, I could not get that last remaining bit of dried blood out of it—it was as if it had been painted on. Then there was a knock at the door.

You can't see directly into the kitchen from the front door, so I wasn't worried until I heard Smithy's mother's voice.

*Oh no, I can't let her see me like this; she thinks I am one of the few decent people hanging around with her son*, I thought.

Panicked, I ran into the garage with the syringe and rushed to put the lid on; at that moment, my fingers slipped and the tip of the needle went straight into the top of my index finger. A surprising amount of blood flowed for a good ten minutes while I hid in the main bathroom until she left.

A few nights after the dirty-syringe episode, Smithy was listening to triple j loudly in the lounge room. For the most part, the biggest threat, as perceived in my psychosis, was the radio—particularly triple j. I would think that Smithy was texting them and telling them what I was doing, that the songs were about me, and that the presenters on the radio were doing impersonations of me.

On the Friday night at the end of the same week, Smithy had two female visitors to the house, who had visited before. After they left, I started to wonder if they were who they said they were. Why were they so worried? Were they actually relatives of mine who had been sent in to see if I was okay?

While I was sitting there thinking about this, Smithy walked in, his Popeye-zombie eye flaring again, and said he had given them the last of his meth for free. He did this, apparently, because one of the women had sent him a sext telling him that she and her sister were about to take a bath together.

This text message struck me as being part of their subterfuge, and added to my desire to work out whom they really were. I asked him first if I could text them, and he said no, very angrily, and then I asked if they were prostitutes. The answer was, again, no. Not having my usual capacities to just let things lie, I then asked him—relatively innocently and probably naively—whether he thought that maybe they were winding him up in order to get free crystal meth.

'Are you sure they're not just manipulating you, Smithy? I mean, do these girls ever pay for the drugs you give them?'

'That's none of your fucking business.'

'Well, I just find it highly unlikely that two sisters would get in a bath together, and that the only time they talk sexy to you is when they're half an hour away.'

'Well, nobody wants to fuck *you,* Luke. You smell like shit, and why don't you go and have a look at yourself in the mirror?'

Which, I think, is probably a good opportunity, for the sake of clarity, to explain that I was experiencing a mix of psychotic ideas, clear ideas that were based on fact, and things I was not, and am still not, completely sure about.

## My psychotic ideas

- There was a paedophile ring in town being run out of the Coffee Club.
- My ex Nathaniel had been turned into a woman who now visited the house.
- I had been chosen to become a famous music performer.
- Smithy and my parents had been trying to kill me.
- Everything I had been seeing on Facebook was about me in secret codes.
- People from other countries were communicating with me via telepathy.
- People were talking about me on the radio and television in a nasty way.

### Things I wasn't sure about

- Was Smithy trying to get me to do things sexually while I was off my face, even though I told him no?
- How upset was Beck about this sexual attention? Did she feel she'd become a third wheel in the friendship?
- How many times did Nathaniel cheat on me that I did not know about, and did Smithy ever come on to him?
- How damaged were the kids by all of this, and how much did they understand about what was going on?
- Were these women manipulating Smithy to get drugs off him?
- Was using crystal meth making me more creative? Or was I destroying my brain? Or both?
- Had I been the victim of a lot of bad things in my life, or did I have a persecution complex?
- Was I actually on some kind of Journey, or was this all due to psychosis?

All of this was floating around my head on this night, and I guess — as psychotics do — I had a need to weave it all together so that it made some kind of sense. As I was doing that, a guy named Jake — who was a frequent visitor to the house — knocked on the door, came right in, and sat on the bed next to Smithy. His talk eventually moved to a pretty blonde 16-year-old girl he'd seen in the house, and he complained about how unfair he thought it was that sex with younger teenagers was unlawful, before launching into a story about his own sexual experiences, at the age of twelve, with his neighbours, in their thirties at the time.

I wasn't sure whether he was joking or making it up or what, but I left the room. In the garage, trying to put it out of my mind, I started writing poems. I couldn't stop thinking that there was something going on, though, and this led to me thinking about the Coffee Club paedophile ring, and Nathaniel, and I had this urgent feeling that there was a secret for me to uncover.

Why was Smithy constantly talking about sex? Why was he constantly masturbating in front of me, even though I didn't want him to? There seemed to be a kind of conspiracy, and then it hit me: one night, years and years ago, my ex John was visiting on the same night as Nathaniel. We were lying in Beck's bed watching a horror movie, when Nathaniel left the room because he was scared. When I got up the next day, there was a strange vibe around the house: looking back on it now, I was convinced that all four of them had slept in the lounge room, and that John and Nathaniel had taken turns having sex with Smithy. I even believed they had given me a sleeping tablet to make it happen. Then when Nathaniel dumped me, Smithy kicked me out of Beck's house, and all this so he could turn Nathaniel into a transsexual and keep sleeping with him. It all made a terrible kind of sense, and so I said to Smithy, straight out, 'Why did you sleep with Nathaniel?'

He looked at me, and I looked at him. He seemed puzzled, and I stood over him as he sat on his bed; I looked at his soft, supple neck and his eye sockets, and I felt my elbows and my fingers and my fists, and I wondered: *How could he have done this to me? How could he have told Nathaniel to break up with me just so he could turn him into a transsexual to satisfy his weird sexual appetites?* I could imagine Smithy whispering about it to Nathaniel when I went to sleep.

'I finally worked out what you've been up to,' I said. 'Nathaniel dumped me at the same time you guys stopped talking to me—this all seems a bit convenient to me.'

He was looking at me curiously, guiltily; he had even stopped masturbating.

'How could you do this to me?' I asked.

'Do what?' he replied. And the more I asked, and the more I stood over him, and the closer I got, the more he looked scared and ashamed, and started checking out the window as if he thought I might have a gang waiting for him outside.

And so I moved closer, ready to attack, and I said: 'For the last time, why did you fuck Nathaniel?'

On that he stood up, raced towards me unexpectedly, and said, 'Don't you fucking threaten me, you piece of shit. I could beat the living fuck out of you without even trying.' I went from homicidal to terrified of being killed in an instant, and in that same instant, I realised I was being paranoid and that I had upset him.

By then he'd kicked me out of his room, but I became confused. I couldn't remember what had just happened or why he had closed the door or why he was angry. I felt terribly lonely standing there outside his door; I wondered if he *had* tried to kill me, and I really, really felt like a bong. I called through the closed door, 'Please, Smithy, you are the only person I have left in my life, please let me in.'

'Fuck off,' he said, and upon hearing this I felt deeply wounded, and scared. He could easily crush my face in if he wanted to.

'Please, Smithy, I'm sorry, I feel suicidal because of what happened.'

'I don't have to put up with this fucking shit from you, Luke.'

'What shit?'

He opened the door slightly so I could just see his face and said, '*Stop stealing my fucking pot.* I know you've been stealing it for months on end.'

I walked outside to an unremarkable grey day, the cold wind tingling my skin, and started thinking again that maybe it *was* possible that Smithy had slept with Nathaniel, that maybe he shut the door because he was guilty.

After wandering in circles for hours, I got on the train and headed for the local hospital; I didn't have a Myki card, but when the woman at the gate saw the expression on my face, she opened the gate and said, 'I hope you're okay'. Otherwise I don't remember the train trip, and I don't remember walking to the hospital.

But I do remember walking into the hospital, into an empty emergency waiting room with hard white floors. I remember telling the woman at reception that I needed help. The woman was meek and mild, and told me to take a seat. Not long after, I was taken into a small windowless room with a man who appeared to be a typical nerd, apart from the full-sleeve tattoos on both arms. He asked me a range of questions, looking at me with dark eyes and through dark glasses, about what I had been doing, what I had been thinking about, why I was doing what I was doing. For the first time in a very long time I remembered what I really was doing: 'I moved into the house to research a story. I'm a journalist; I just got a bit too caught up in it.' He told me he also used to be a journalist, for a small regional newspaper in England, and he asked me what I had been doing for money. I explained that I had still been working, and he asked me who for, how much they paid me, and how often I wrote for them. The answer seemed to annoy him in some way, and he told me that I didn't need to see a doctor because I was still functional, and if I didn't suffer from psychosis outside of meth use, I needed to see a drug counsellor not a doctor.

'I've been here before,' I told him. 'A few years ago, I came when I was clean and feeling suicidal and you let me stay—'

He cut in: 'Yes, I know, I have the notes here.'

He asked what the hospital could do for me, and I said I didn't know. He gave me a card and told me to go to a drug counselling drop-in service, which wouldn't be open for another two days. When I asked for a Valium, his response was 'We're not giving you any more drugs'. He told me there was nothing they could do for me, and left the room. I returned to the admissions desk and told them that I felt suicidal. I was finally admitted, but then doctor after doctor came up to tell me there was nothing they could do for me and that I had to leave. I believe I was obviously in need of help — I was talking to myself and experiencing some mildly psychotic delusions (such as telling staff that my mum had dementia and telling triage I had been communicating with people via telepathy) mixed with moments of genuine clarity. I had been feeling suicidal all morning, and the hospital was the only place for me. The doctors I saw told me that being in the hospital was making my condition worse, and that there was nothing they could do. I know this might seem a bit unbelievable — that I could be begging for help in that state and the medical staff refused to help — but turning away suicidal and psychotic patients, especially drug-affected ones, is a surprisingly common problem in Australian hospitals.

In retrospect, it's not clear why the hospital didn't simply provide me with a low dose of anti-psychotics and keep me for observation (as the relevant methamphetamine treatment guidelines suggest a health-care worker should do). It is tempting to conclude that the staff lacked experience and expertise in dealing with those experiencing crystal-meth-induced agitation (and weren't trained on the relevant guidelines); however, there have been a number of cases reported by the Victorian coroners court and by plaintiff law firms that show that several people have committed suicide or assaulted somebody after being released from the hospital I visted, in some cases while still showing signs of psychosis.

There are a number of ways of looking at this issue. First and foremost is the lack of access to mental-health services within the community, which means people suffering acute psychological distress often end up in under-resourced emergency rooms full of medical staff with no formal training in mental-health care. The local drug-counselling centre that the staff referred me to wasn't open until Monday (I was at the hospital on a Saturday).

Second, many people who come to a hospital emergency room feeling suicidal have reported that they don't feel they are treated adequately, and sometimes not even treated respectfully. In December 2014, the mental-health advocacy group Sane Australia released a report they conducted with the University of New South Wales. The report was based on interviews with 31 Australians who had made attempts on their own life. Eighty per cent of those interviewed reported that their hospital experience was 'negative', and a third of the study sample felt their concerns were not taken seriously. *The Guardian* Australia covered the release of the report, and quoted Patrick McGorry: '[I]t is all too common that the patient who made an attempt on their life, who is desperate and in emotional pain, turns up and is seen by emergency-department staff as a nuisance rather than as someone with a life-threatening emergency.'

Third, people who experience both mental illness and drug addiction frequently fall through service gaps because they don't quite fit either category. Surveys from the Australian Injecting and Illicit Drug Users League in 2011 found that of a 300-person sample of illicit-drug users, 60 per cent of them said they had experienced discrimination at a hospital, making it the second most likely site of discrimination after police stations. I had attended this hospital previously, in 2009, when I was feeling suicidal, and I was given an anti-psychotic and allowed to stay the night. I was also given counselling. When I arrived on drugs, I was — and I hate to say this — more or less told to fuck off.

Fourth, medical and hospital staff can tend towards 'black-and-white' thinking and be incredibly defensive about the quality of their care. Several mental-health rights groups have told me it is common that after a complaint is made by a mental-health patient, the hospital will buckle down and go into legal adversarial mode: denying that anything is wrong with the system, or that they made any sort of mistake, be it individual or systemic. And why is this? It's possible that it happens because a mentally unwell complainant is unlikely to be believed no matter how legitimate their complaints. On the release of the Sane Australia report, Sally McCarthy, an associate professor and the immediate past president of the Australasian College for Emergency Medicine, said that complaints about the standard of psychiatric care in emergency departments were 'ignorant'.

When I eventually complained to the hospital about my treatment, not only did they deny that staff had done anything wrong, but the hospital also said—and this despite the obvious fact that I was on crystal meth, as demonstrated by their referral for me to go a drug-counselling centre—that 'there was no evidence' I was affected by crystal meth at the time. They also implied that I pretended to be suicidal just so I could stay in the hospital. It appears that rather than attempt to fix problems, hospitals instead throw money at lawyers and law firms, and work from the point of view that a mentally unwell patient is unreliable as a witness.

On the night in question, confused about why I'd left Smithy's house and no longer sure of exactly what had occurred, I went back there, and went to bed.

When I got up the next day, my mind had once again changed direction—I was feeling scared again, too scared to leave my bedroom, so I texted Beck about what had happened, but she never texted back. Another day passed, which I spent in the library, and when I got home, Smithy glared at me, deliberately and savagely. Feeling unsafe, and paranoid that he was plotting something, I asked a friend, Sarah, if I could stay at her place for the night. She said yes, so I hopped on a train.

When the train rolled into Noble Park, I got a message from

Sarah that said: 'Sorry babe, I wish I could help you, but tonight isn't a good night'. 'Sarah, I have nowhere else to go, I am scared to go home'; 'Just not tonight, me and David are breaking up', and so I got off the train, and now I wasn't so much scared as just plain furious.

The short winter day had come to an end, and I started to feel cold and scared. I had about $50 left. It was dark, and I was convinced that Smithy wanted to kill me, and this time I believed he had friends who were waiting at his house to do it. I rang my parents, but the combination of my drug-induced psychosis and what I perceived as their indifference to my plight was a toxic one. After a series of increasingly aggressive calls, my parents stopped answering their phones.

By the time I got back to Smithy's, it was nearly 11.00pm. Beck and Smithy had been discussing something; it seemed that there was a kind of peace or closeness between them. Beck said she wanted to talk to me about something, and we went for a drive. Once in the car, she began defending Smithy against the accusations of various women who'd said he'd been touching them inappropriately, or harassing them by text. I tried to stay as neutral as I could, but my own experience told me there was something in what these women were saying. Eventually, Beck got to the point: Smithy had accused me of stealing his pot, and wanted me out of the house. The ensuing fight escalated to the point where I punched the dashboard, and she threw me out of the car. When I'd walked back to Smithy's, I found them cuddled together on the couch.

I snuck into my bedroom, packed my things, and snuck out the back door. I took my suitcase to the local high school, made myself a makeshift bed, and settled down to sleep.

*Perhaps I can just live like this*, I thought. *No illusions, no walls, no people, no stupid dreams; I can just survive like a wild animal.* The next day, I hid my suitcase, and stole chocolate from

Kmart. I had no money left. Then the next night came, and it was far colder. I was so tired, but I couldn't sleep; every time I did manage to have a micro-sleep, I dreamt about being close to a fire, but the fire kept going out. When I woke up I was freezing, and I realised that this was a terrible idea.

I wanted warmth so badly I felt as if I could knock on a stranger's door. I plucked up the courage to ask my estranged ex if I could stay with him in his dilapidated terrace house in Footscray. Much to my surprise, he agreed and was now a chronic meth-head himself. He lived with a guy named Sammy, also called Mr Sheen, a frankly terrifying human being. Mr Sheen was built like a brick shithouse; he was a big-time steroid user, and old-school intravenous ice user, and it was no surprise to me to hear he had spent time in both jail and a psych ward.

One night Mr Sheen cracked, like, really cracked. He was cleaning when he told me I was not allowed to leave my ex's room. 'You're dirty,' he told me. 'You're spreading germs around the house.' When he caught me going to the toilet at 5.00am, he lit up an angry red and started screaming in my face: 'Get the fuck out now, you dirty fucking cunt—I'll fucking bash the fuck out of you.'

So I left, wandering around South Yarra for a while before heading for the train station, which even at 6.00am had government-hired 'protective officers' hanging about. With nowhere else to go, I returned to Pakenham, where I sat by a big lake carved out of the wetlands, a sheet of mist sitting on the top, and started to cry, thinking, 'I need to go the police'.

## Chapter Fourteen

# Bundaberg

'THIS STATEMENT IS off the record,' a male officer at the Pakenham police station told me in a small, windowless interview room. 'Nothing you will say will be used to implicate you in any crime. This is just a chat between us.'

And I told them everything that happened.

'So, what about you? Where are you at now?' another officer asked.

'I have nowhere to live, nowhere to go; I have no money, and I've been sleeping rough.'

'What about your parents?' he asked.

'I abused them, I threatened to kill them, they want nothing to do with me.'

'You're welcome to ring them now and tell them where you are,' he told me.

So I did, and Dad answered. Straightaway I said, 'I am sorry, I don't know what came over me.'

'That's alright, mate, we're relieved you're back to yourself—I'll put Mum on.'

Mum answered and I apologised to her as well; she echoed Dad's sentiment that they were glad to have me back to normal.

But I still didn't have anywhere to stay. So I went to a friend's house, where I stayed for a few nights. In the meantime, I emailed Mum and told her I had nowhere to go; she suggested a rehab, then a homeless shelter, and then my uncle's house. I rang her one night to ask her if I could come back and live with them while I recovered, but she said she didn't feel safe around me after phone calls I had made, and emails I had sent—which I actually don't even remember sending (though it turns out I did)—saying that I hated her and I wished she were dead.

The conversation ended abruptly, and I went to stay with my schizophrenic uncle, who also lived in Pakenham—a charming character who would interrupt my story of what had happened every time I mentioned a female to ask what her breasts looked like. After two days, he rang my dad to say he didn't want me living with him anymore, because my clothes stank. So I had to ring Mum again; this time, I agreed with everything she said, because I did not fancy sleeping outside in the winter, and not long after, I was on a plane back to sunny Bundaberg.

And then there I was: I had the sunshine, and my books, and the gyms, and the time to try to work out where it so wrong. 'I fucked up' was the simplest answer. Yet 'I fucked up again, aged thirty-four, with two university degrees under my belt and a world of opportunity ahead of me, all the while believing I was on a mystical journey, and had to move back home to live with my parents in central Queensland' raised some serious questions.

That said, under the circumstances that preceded my escape, quitting meth wasn't actually that hard—in fact, it was a relief. The possession passed quickly and painlessly, even joyously. I got to my parents' house at the best time of the year: winter. It was a relief not to be surrounded by unpredictable meth-heads; to have my own bed, and to be left alone to do my own thing. I felt happy. Maybe it's as simple as that I was sick to death of taking the drug, and of everything that went with it, by the time I arrived in Bundaberg. I would write in *The Saturday Paper* just a few weeks after I quit:

> For me, my foray into meth showed that liberalism has its limits. I learnt that meth use is not merely a transgressive and misunderstood rebellion against the pressures of working life and the banality of Australian suburbia. It does kill, and when it doesn't it can be almost Faustian when taken in large doses.
>
> I say almost because meth doesn't take away people's 'souls' — the drug delivers self-centered hedonism. Many addicts have often told me life can't compare to the pleasure the drug provides. But meth can never deliver the things that make us tick.

So I can admit I was feeling pretty damn good. But the longer my recovery lasted, the more I started to believe that not only I had developed an insatiable itch which I really needed to scratch, but I recognised that I wasn't feeling much of *anything* if I wasn't itchy, which caused me to wonder: *Being itchy is better than not feeling anything at all, isn't it?*

According to former addict and author Joseph Sharp, the best thing an addict can do in the first month after getting off crystal meth is to eat, hydrate, take vitamins, and eat some more. In this way, the initial recovery period can be enjoyable; you can gorge yourself on food knowing you are not going to put on any weight, and you can often do nothing except look after yourself. Everyone tends to be extra nice to you during this period, because they are so glad you quit, which also helps. Sharp says the first eight weeks of crystal meth can actually be a bit of a 'honeymoon period' where the crash has lifted, and you get a little natural high as you restore yourself to optimal physical health. Then after this honeymoon period, about forty-five days in to sobriety, you hit a 'seemingly insurmountable Wall of depression, boredom and despair'.

Dr Nicole Lee told me that one of the biggest problems ice addicts face is that because crystal meth releases so much dopamine, it makes it hard for recovering users and abusers to experience pleasure in everyday life. She said that many users don't just run out of dopamine, they actually destroy their dopamine receptors, which means that their bodies can no longer produce it. It can take twelve to eighteen months before those systems are functioning again.

Poor thinking habits, as well as paranoia, that were created during long crystal-meth sessions can linger, too; when you come out of the fog of drug addiction, you find new wounds and pains and obsessions, and re-discover old ones, as well as focus on age-old questions of meaning and purpose. When you're on crystal meth, or in psychosis, these problems can seem abstract and exciting—but once you stop using, life can seem predictable, slow, and dull.

In the aftermath, I not only had the feeling that nothing was quite hitting the spot, but also the struggle to re-make a narrative for my life when the old one had almost been wiped clean. After six weeks had passed, I began to have recurring memories about my exclusion in high school which cut and re-cut me over and over: the teachers who told me to leave school because my written work was 'so crap'; the fact that my creative flourishes were constantly treated as medical and disciplinary issues at home and at school (I had compulsory counselling at high school because I wrote freaky short stories and gave them to other students); getting kicked out of home shortly thereafter, and my mother's persistent denial of those events. For months on end, one angry thought lead to another, until they all seemed interrelated and all had the same cause: I had been wronged—and now there was no escape hatch, no eject button.

There are some 'simple' theories of addiction: *negative reinforcement*—drug use can become addictive because withdrawal causes dysphoria; *positive reinforcement*—people take drugs because they like using them; and *incentive salience*—drug use is caused by cravings caused by the drug-induced sensitisation of brain systems. Addiction is generally thought to stem from a complex relationship between genes, environment, one's upbringing, and life trauma. People who have a mental illness are, for instance, far more likely to develop an addiction than those who do not. One increasingly popular theory is *disease theory*, which suggests drug addiction is the result of biology, but even that idea has come under scrutiny lately: Dr Marc Lewis argues in his book *The Biology of Desire: why addiction is not a disease* that addiction is a behavioural problem that requires willpower and motivation to change.

Dr Carl Hart suggests drug addiction may be related to social opportunity. Hart watched relatives become crack addicts living in squalor and stealing from their mothers, and observed childhood friends ending up in prisons and morgues. Dr Hart says his research shows that people in poor communities have fewer 'competing reinforces' to provide them pleasure and gratification, thus leading many people to choose drugs through lack of opportunity, and leading him to what we might recognise as a rather familiar-sounding left-liberal conclusion on drug abuse:

> What I now know is that the drugs themselves are not the real problem. The real problems are: poverty, unemployment, selective drug law enforcement, ignorance, and the dismissal of science surrounding these drugs.

Another potentially complementary theory, advanced by Harvard psychiatrist Edward J. Khantzian, says that drug addicts typically show a profound inability to calm and soothe themselves when stressed. Furthermore, many drug addicts tend to have had mothers, and no doubt many fathers, whom they describe as 'relatively cold, unresponsive, and under protective', and who, despite seeming to be very interested in their child's performance, send very mixed messages when it comes to celebrating their achievements. On the other hand, the far-right 'moral model' of addiction theory presupposes that drug abusers are morally deficient and need to be punished for their use of illicit drugs.

During my recovery at my parents' house, the Victorian parliamentary inquiry into crystal meth delivered its very extensive two-part report, stating first and foremost that while most people who use methamphetamine don't need intensive treatment, when treatment was required, there were a number of interventions that had been shown to work: brief interventions; cognitive behaviour therapy (CBT); acceptance and commitment therapy (ACT); motivational enhancement; contingency management; and residential rehabilitation.

The report also said that many working on the frontline had a lack of expertise in the area of crystal-methamphetamine use, and that many frontline agencies reported feeling pessimistic about their ability to treat crystal-meth addicts. This isn't uncommon, though: professor of criminal justice at Illinois State University Ralph Weisheit writes in his book *Methamphetamine: its history, pharmacology, and treatment* that pessimism about treatments for a problem drug is often prevalent in the early and peak stages of a drug surge. His review of research showed that about 50 per cent of crystal-meth addicts remained clean for twelve months after completing a residential treatment—about the same rate as for other drugs.

Research by Rebecca McKetin compared 248 former crystal-meth users treated in a rehabilitation program, 112 in a detox program, and 101 meth users who weren't undergoing any treatment at the time, but were still attempting to give up the drug. Over a three-year period, McKetin and her researchers estimated that rehab resulted in 48 per cent of people remaining abstinent from the drug, compared to 15 per cent in the other groups. This tallies with research undertaken by health journalist and former alcoholic Anne Fletcher. In her spectacularly comprehensive book *Inside Rehab: the surprising truth about addiction treatment and how to get help that works*, she details the high dropout rates of rehab, reporting that 40–60 per cent of those who complete a program end up relapsing. Alcoholic Anonymous' rates are even lower, she says, with some studies showing that just 10 per cent of people who go through the program stay clean.

One gets the sense that many of us, even the experts, are still very much learning about what works for all sorts of drug addictions. Perhaps this is because for so long, drug addiction was treated as a crime or a type of vagrancy (perhaps it still is in an indirect sense), and so medical treatment approaches don't have a particularly long history. And, given that they are medical approaches, they tend to focus on the individual rather than on the social or cultural factors surrounding them. One also gets the feeling that nobody really knows yet what the best approach to drug addiction is. Many people regard drug use as a simple choice, and drug addiction as a moral failing. On the other hand, drug use is also the domain of celebrities and artists — making it seem vaguely glamorous, and even an assertion of autonomy and identity in some circumstances.

And as crystal meth is a relatively recent drug, particularly in Australia, individual treatment solutions are still in their early stages. Along with a lack of rehab services (discussed in detail in Chapter 15) many professionals are unsure of the best way to treat crystal-meth addicts. As a result, many recovering addicts are writing their own scripts about how best to recover, with varying results.

I had been through rehab before and it helped, but ultimately it didn't work; one of the mistakes I made was believing that once the 'problem drug' was gone, then most of my other problems would also disappear. I learnt the benefits of exercise, reading, helping others, and getting fully absorbed into doing something that I loved—but things still had this bitter taste, and there were ripple effects from my time in the house that seemed as if they would never still.

Then came my book deal, this wonderful book deal, and somehow it seemed that my struggles had managed to fulfil a purpose. Many people suddenly found me fascinating and insightful, and I was contacted by national media outlets from all over the country.

In the weeks after I moved to Bundaberg, I had hoped that Nathaniel and I might be able to rekindle our relationship. I sent him seven emails telling him how much I missed him, and that I was worried about him. After six weeks of not replying, he sent an email asking, 'Do you have any money I can have?'

Beck had not responded to any of my messages since I left the house, and was reportedly very angry I was writing this book. My mum initially seemed pleased, but soon took to Facebook, linking to my article in *The Saturday Paper* and sharing details of my life that I felt breached my privacy.

I was also fielding calls from Stacey, Beck's sister, in which she said, 'I've seen what is going on Luke, and I know you've seen what is going on. I'm going to ring child protection and I think you should do the same.'

She told me that Beck had continued using crystal meth right through the winter and deep into the spring, as well as the never-ending iPad game-playing that went with it. The arguments between her and Smithy worsened as Beck became increasingly worried that he was seeing another woman, and that she might be missing out on her share of meth. One day, things boiled over—a stoush started when they were both coming down, and both at their worst. Things got physical, and Smithy hit Beck in the mouth right in front of Alice.

At one stage, Beck sat outside Smithy's house, screaming and tooting the horn for over an hour. She had a physical scuffle with one of his housemates out the front, and eventually the neighbours called the police and she was arrested; Smithy would then get an intervention order preventing her from going near him or the twins. Following this, Beck went to stay at her mum's, who became increasingly confused by her changing stories about people getting raped in their house or Smithy gang-banging her friends, or her outbursts about why it was wrong to feed wild birds just an hour after she had been doing it herself.

Stacey kept sending me Facebook messages urging me to go to child protection—but knowing that I was still angry with Beck and Smithy, I said I wanted to wait a bit longer before I made the call.

Amid all this, I decided that with my book advance, I would book a ticket overseas to anywhere—anywhere would be fine—so I picked a flight to Kuala Lumpur for February, the cheapest flight I could find.

I started going on long half-day hikes around town, through bushland, lakeside parks, sugar cane fields, and outlying suburbs of Bundaberg. I walked for hours at a time, counting birds, trying to work out which plants were native and which were introduced, day-dreaming. Every day I would find a new route, or, at least, a new street; one day, when I was walking along the great Burnett River, I took a slight detour and came across a set of buildings in 1970s yellow brick. There must have been seven or eight of them, resembling a small hospital or prison.

There was a sign out of the front: 'Bridges, Drug and Alcohol Centre, Dual Diagnosis Clinic'.

I walked in to see a woman with dark eyes and blonde hair,

who asked for my details as 'What a girl wants, what a girl needs' played in the background. She took me into a small room where I told her my story, and she booked me an appointment. Three days later, I was back at the clinic—to my surprise, my appointment was with the same woman who had been at reception the day I first walked in.

When we sat down, in a much larger interview room, my back to the window, and its view of palm trees, bamboo, and sugar cane, I detected a delightful mix of rattiness and sensitivity about her. She told me her name was Jay, and that she would be looking at the 'underlying issues' that led to my addictive behaviour, and that her therapeutic approach was based largely on CBT—the same therapy that I had undergone during my stay in residential rehab in 2008, and which was designed to help someone identify their 'unhelpful thoughts and behaviours', and to learn or relearn 'healthier skills and habits'.

I relayed what had happened over the past three months, which became a rapid overview of my life: the bullying at high school—how it cost me three years, how I didn't think I would ever heal from it, how my parents failed to protect me—and the failed demo at triple j, which had effectively cost me my first career.

She observed me with concentration as I told the story, and at the end she said: 'I don't want to sound clichéd, Luke, and I do understand some of the things you are talking about. I came from an abusive background and I am a perfectionist—I often just let go altogether when things go wrong—but the one thing that I have learnt, the thing that gets me through, is the ability to take everything bad I have been through, and use it to find my strengths. I've found that if I talk about my strengths, think about my strengths, and concentrate on them, I feel better about myself, and my life gets better.'

She went to say that my negative experiences has also had

positive effects: that they had made me more compassionate, and that the person I was had been formed by my negative experiences. Although this made sense to me, I was also cynical of anything that might seem like a 'lightning bolt' or epiphany, not only because I was distrusting my own brain, but also because I had been through rehab before, and had all these big 'realisations' only to then became a drug abuser again.

One mistake I was determined *not* to repeat from my last rehab was to be overly optimistic about life when I stopped using the drug. After rehab in 2008, I felt as if the world was glowing with goodness by the time I got out. I believed everything depended on me only, that self-responsibility was virtually omnipotent. Then once I got out, I had the same job at the ABC with limited opportunities to work anywhere else; the same nepotism and celebration of mediocrity which drove me to madness; the same lack of affordable housing; 90 per cent of people still frustrated me, and the only people I liked were other drug users. The idea that your life is purely the result of willpower is quite simply at odds with reality. The notion of addiction is, in part, a modern, liberal idea: individual freedom is thought to be potentially limitless, but opportunity and experience will also be limited by economics, talent, practicability, other people, the body, and life in general.

I wanted my beliefs to be *realistic* not convenient. I can't make myself believe in a higher power, fatalism, or the essential goodness of things purely because it might be more psychologically healthy and spiritually fulfilling to do so. Fatalism can leave one dangerously passive. A belief in a higher power can lead to an abrogation of responsibility—and besides, when everything is said and done, I'm just not sure I see the world that way. During my recovery, I often wondered if my addiction would have still been seen as such a problem if I had endless amounts of money, didn't bother anybody, worked a lot, still looked okay, and didn't need anywhere to live.

My adult life has been filled with drug use, and the five years in which I wasn't using weren't especially joy-filled or exciting. My friends of ten, fifteen, twenty years are all drug takers, and many of my friendships have been formed around taking drugs. I have had trouble forming relationships outside of this, finding excitement outside of drugs, and escaping pits of despair even when I'm clean. One possible solution I have considered is to use occasionally, but with that said—that's what I did last time I left rehab, and I believe now that I sold myself short with this approach. I stopped looking forward to things, I stopped pushing myself, I stopped achieving things, I stopped living life to the fullest because I knew I could disappear into a drug world.

In my friendless state in the aftermath of my addiction, the drug seemed to have created an abyss of strange, new needs; it seemed that the crystal palace would never be destroyed, even when its spell was broken. Sociologist Emilé Durkheim says human desire is a bottomless and insatiable pit, and that the world we live in is full of never-ending wants; this leads to 'anomie', which is the breakdown of social bonds between an individual and the community, and which creates a sense of purposelessness.

Stacey kept on emailing me to ask if I was going to ring child protection, and eventually I decided it was probably the right thing to do—it would, at the very least, force Beck and Smithy to get their act together. When I rang, I was transferred to a woman with a thick Indian accent, and I told her pretty much everything you have read about in this book, including my involvement in it. Beck already—for reasons I'm not aware of—had a case manager at the Child Protection Unit (CPU). This case manager kept on pressing me on whether I had colluded with other people who had been to the house to report Beck and Smithy. I told her that I had spoken with Stacey, and that neither of us had any contact with anybody else who had been to the house. As it turned out, three other regular visitors to the house had also reported them to the department. Eventually, a formal investigation was initiated, and both were asked to take drug tests, or risk losing their children.

Not long after the CPU investigation started, Beck stopped taking drugs, and, by all reports, enjoyed the novelty of her sobriety. Smithy refused to take the drug tests. Beck did everything the child-protection department asked her to do. She starting seeing a psychiatrist, and she continued to pass her drug tests. As the investigations continued, however, more pus was found festering just beneath the surface. When they rang Pakenham primary school, they found that Alice—the middle child, who was then in Year 6—had missed nearly a month of school days. Now that they lived in the town, fifteen minutes' drive away from the school, Beck had not been getting up in the morning to take her. When the department spoke with Beck's family, they would tell them that she had been disappearing for days, and sometimes a week at a time, to go to Smithy's—without warning—leaving Alice alone, and without a lift to school. When Beck *did* come back, she was usually so tired she would sleep for two or three days at a times, leaving it to her mother to cook and clean for Alice. The department would eventually make an order that it was Beck's mum's responsibility to take Alice to school.

I kept seeing my counsellor, Jay, who told me that part of the overwhelming emotion I was experiencing was that I was 'catching up' on my feelings. Using drugs had numbed me, and now I had a lot of repressed emotion that needed to find expression.

I agreed that it might be that, but I felt there were also things I was legitimately angry about. I found it a bit too neat to reduce all my experiences to things that 'made me stronger' or 'happened for a reason'.

We moved on to talking about how my desire for meth was going. I told her I had been experiencing intense cravings.

'How strong?'

'Pretty strong.'

'Does the thought of using ever make you drool with excitement?'

'Sometimes, yes.'

'Have you been considering using again?'

'Um, yes, I think if I go down to Melbourne again, and see some old friends, if I just have it once, it won't matter and I might actually—'

'I thought so.'

'Why do you say that?

'You're self-victimising, Luke. I've seen it time and time again: when somebody is having cravings for drugs, they begin to paint a picture of themselves as being a victim, so they feel they deserve to have meth. "Just one more shot, once won't hurt"—these are the kinds of thoughts people have before they relapse. You are responsible, Luke, and the more you realise this, the more empowered you will feel.'

I need to mention here that during the time I was in Bundaberg, I was sentenced to a hundred and fifty hours of community service for spitting on a café employee who had asked me to stop eating food I'd bought elsewhere on the café premises. I was very sorry about what I'd done—it was out of character—but I had been humiliated by what I perceived as the employee's aggression towards me. Needless to say, the court case went against me, and although I accepted that what I had done was wrong, I appealed against the ruling, as I desperately wanted to get overseas. My appeal was denied, though, and so I was obligated to stay in Bundaberg until I'd finished my community service hours.

I found the environment toxic—on my first day, I was offered crystal meth and marijuana, as well as being harassed for being gay. I just wanted to get out of Bundaberg, but I couldn't. That night, I told Mum I needed to go the psych ward and left the house. I walked in circles around the streets, with no shoes on, forgetting where I was going or what I was doing; I kept having visions of cutting myself. When I got back to the house, I snuck back in to see that Mum was still sitting there playing her computer game. I told her how much I hated living with her because it was impossible to hold a conversation with her. I became increasingly out of control as I told her that I knew she and Dad had been discussing the 'spitting incident' in judgemental, non-constructive terms, and that neither had offered the slightest bit of help or support or advice. I went on to attack her personally, as all my frustration and the resentment of years spilled out of me.

After I'd calmed down, I rang Lifeline and spoke to them for half an hour. I then slept for twelve hours, and when I woke up, Mum came into the room looking as if she hadn't slept all night. She told me that she was tired of my abuse, and that I had to leave immediately or she would call the police. I said she was playing the victim. She in turn told me that she felt 'threatened' because I was in the house, and so I left the house and sent her an email asking her if I could just stay until I got the rest of my book advance.

To which she responded:

01/02/2015
From: J Williams
Luke I would like you leave tonight. I would prefer we do this without police involvement.

http://www.bundabergtouristpark.com.au/

http://oakwoodvanpark.com.au/

http://bundyregionconnect.qld.gov.au/24-hour-crisis-support/bundaberg-homeless-mens-hostel

Everything is packed and ready.


01/02/2015
From: Luke Williams
Okay thanks.


When I got back, Dad asked where I was going, and I explained I would be sleeping rough for at least one night because I didn't have enough money to stay in the homeless shelter. I asked him to drive me to Bridges (the drug and counselling centre), where I slept on the porch, under cover, with a view to the stars and the palm trees, on a spectacular night during which the temperature did not drop below 26 degrees. There were crickets creaking and bats screeching, and patches of thin wind-cloud over the moon, which looked about as comfortable as a mattress starts to seem after two hours of lying on concrete. In the morning, I was woken by a woman with glasses as I lay in the bright morning sunshine on a towel and a pillow.

'Is Jay here?' I asked.

'She will be soon. Don't worry, love, we will get you sorted,' she said 'Do you want a shower?'

'Yes.'

'A coffee?'

'Yes.'

After the shower, Jay came in, and tears welled in her eyes when I told her what had happened; this was the first time I had seen her since before the sentencing.

Jay referred me to a social worker, who said I was a 'high needs, complex client'. The social worker gave me food vouchers, paid for me to stay in a cheap motel room, and told me again and again how much she enjoyed my company — a small kindness on a horrible day.

The motel room was small and hot, and my window had a

lovely view to the KFC next door. But how could I *really* feel angry with people, and angry at a society, when getting help when I was down and out was so easy?

Around the corner from the motel was a particularly beautiful part of town. A reminder that no matter how one feels, whether one is happy, sad, addicted, homeless, high, sober, alone, or in love—some things about the world will always exist whether we are able to see them or not. If we try hard enough we find selflessness, imagination, nature, long walks, a community, good people, and a place where we can pretty much do, or, at least, think whatever we like. There is a massive, wonderful, complex world that exists well outside of me, and what I might be in the mood to perceive.

As I stood by the great flood-prone Burnett River, which has flowed through these parts for hundreds of thousands of years, I felt a breeze that was cool and fresh and easterly—and it kind of smelt like the ocean. I looked up across perfect blue sky that seemed to go on forever. There were at least a hundred different plants before me: patches of old dry eucalypt, regenerated rainforest that ran along a creek, a single tall palm tree dwarfing the lush scrub around it. Moths scattered as I walked, crickets buzzed, lorikeets screeched, there was a gentle buzz of traffic on a busy four-lane highway—I had no idea where it began or finished. I looked up into the sky again as three black waterfowl floated delicately over my head. Half a dozen galahs glided by to land in a rare flowering eucalypt tree, whose smell reminded me that I am but a guest in this wondrous, ancient land, and ultimately a servant to its laws. And one day nothing more than food to help the trees grow their flowers for the birds to suckle. I noticed a massive bird of prey—perhaps a kite or sea eagle—flying around in circles, higher and higher, until I could no longer see it amid the blue. No ordinary bird would fly that high; it moved effortlessly in a vertical direction, all the while maintaining perfect grace and poetry. The further I looked into the sky, the more birds I could see — birds you wouldn't notice unless you stared for a long time, as I was doing. I had no answers, I had no revelations, I had no real plans other than going overseas, I had no idea what I was going to do, or where I was going to live, or what was going to happen, or whether I would find anybody worth loving again. Yet at that moment, the universe was infinite, and my possibilities alive and endless. I guess there was not just possibility but also hope. There will always be light, and whatever light is, is light.

## Chapter Fifteen

# Two steps forward, one step back

I RETURNED TO Melbourne four weeks before I was due to leave for Kuala Lumpur. I decided to work on a project I'd been planning for quite some time — to move into Australia's most notoriously dangerous boarding house, The Gatwick in St Kilda. The Gatwick is a spooky old mansion on Fitzroy Street, a privately owned hostel that gives shelter to 90-odd people at any one time who can't find anywhere else to live: the mentally ill, sex workers, the Indigenous and indigent, the drifters and yes, the drug addicts. I had wanted to write a live-in piece about The Gatwick for a long time. I felt my experience with drug addiction, mental-health problems, and homelessness gave me unique insight, and a unique position from which to understand life for The Gatwick's residents.

It was also a good time, in practical terms, to stay there. I had four weeks to fill before heading Malaysia, and finding a room for a short period of time would have been tricky. I had nothing keeping me in Bundaberg, and after going public with my psychotic episodes and drug addiction in *The Saturday Paper,* I didn't feel comfortable asking anybody if I could stay with them.

One of the major issues I identified that the residents face is boredom. They don't have jobs, they don't play any sport and, in the end, for most of them, there really isn't much to do but find drugs and get high. Most of the Gatwick crew live lives of intense highs and lows, moving from Centrelink paydays to dry days, with nothing much of what many of us would consider to be a meaningful life in between.

I was still not using, and so, with an increasingly clear head, it seemed like a good time to investigate 'Crystal Meth: the policy problem'.

From the very outset, the issue that stood out again and again was a lack of treatment services for people seeking help, and a lack of expertise about crystal-meth treatment among staff in both private and public health institutions. Robyn Reeves, chief executive officer of the Ballarat Community Health Centre, told the Victorian parliamentary inquiry: 'Currently there are no detox facilities apart from some youth detox throughout the entire Grampians region, and the same thing applies for rehabilitation services, so we have staff spending a great deal of time transporting people around the state.'

Debbie Stoneman from Latrobe Community Health Services also told the inquiry: 'When we look at hospital admissions for withdrawal, we are limited in this region to be able to admit a person to a local hospital primarily for a withdrawal, and of course beds are at such a premium that often we cannot keep people in hospital long enough anyway to get through a withdrawal.'

Kit-e Kline from Wathaurong Aboriginal Co-operative also highlighted the lengthy waiting list: 'For me to get someone into detox at the moment is about a six-week wait. That is what you are looking at. Then there could be a three-month wait on rehabilitation. There is definitely a lack of services.'

A lack of drug treatment services appears to be a national problem.

Writing about the New South Wales situation to the federal

parliamentary Joint Committee on Law Enforcement's Inquiry into Crystal Methamphetamine, which was initiated in March 2015, Matt Noffs told the inquiry:

> Our hospitals, psychiatric facilities, and jails are full. Adult drug treatment services such as the Stimulant Treatment program at St Vincent's Hospital, Sydney are full. The economic (not to mention social) implications of intervening in the lives of ice users only after their addiction has become ingrained is enormous.

The South Australian Network of Drug and Alcohol Services told the federal inquiry:

> Funding for Alcohol and Drug treatment services at a Commonwealth level is inadequate and uncertain. Individuals who are not able to receive treatment create a further cost burden on health, policing, and correctional systems.

Mission Australia also told the federal inquiry that the lack of treatment services was of 'urgent priority' because:

> The absence of appropriate detoxification facilities, particularly for young people, remains a considerable barrier to effective interventions and treatment. When a person with ice use is motivated to seek change, appropriate detoxification and rehabilitation facilities need to be available to capitalise on what is often a narrow window of opportunity.

An SBS *Insight* program broadcast in October 2015 featured a former user named Jay, who said he waited three to six months, and called dozens before he could find a rehab. Additionally, Sharon Mestern from Odyssey House in New South Wales told the program that 'we actually have a waiting list to call people back'. A few weeks earlier, SBS *Dateline* broadcast a story showing that an increasing number of Australians are opting to travel to Thailand for immediate treatment rather than joining the waiting list for rehab at home. The story quoted Simon Mott from Thailand's Hope Rehab Centre: 'I need to be grateful to the Australian government for not providing adequate treatment … We've been able to build a strong foundation of having a lot of clients come from Australia'.

In one sense, it's not particularly difficult to work out why there is a lack of government-funded services for crystal-meth addicts. In 2011, Alison Ritter at NDARC put together a remarkable study quantifying how Australian governments spend their drug-related expenditure. She found that over 2009–10, federal and state governments spent a total of $1.7 billion in direct response to illicit-drug use including:

- $1.12 billion on law enforcement — two-thirds of the total spend (66 per cent)
- $361 million on treatment — just over one-fifth (21 per cent)
- $157 million on prevention — just under one-tenth (9 per cent)
- $36 million on harm reduction — 2 per cent

State and territory government spending accounted for more than two thirds of the spend (69 per cent). Moreover, it is state governments who tip the balance of funding, because they are responsible for law-and-order spending, and because a 'tough' approach to law-and-order issues has become an increasingly bipartisan stance from state governments over the past decade.

In the lead up to the election his party eventually won, then Victorian opposition leader, Daniel Andrews, said those caught spreading recipes for ice, or who turned a blind eye to it being sold and used on their premises, would face up to twenty-five years in jail under proposed law changes. He said that harsher penalties would also apply to anyone caught trafficking the drug into or near a primary or secondary school. The New South Wales state government brought in laws so that lower-level ice dealers would get harsher sentences in September 2015, meaning carrying 500 grams, rather than 1 kilogram of crystal meth, as had been the case previously, would now count as a 'large commercial quantity'. A person carrying between 500 grams and 1 kilogram could now face life imprisonment, rather than the maximum 20-year sentence that had been previously available. The New South Wales government also made public announcements asking people to report anybody to the police who they suspected of making or dealing crystal meth. This followed a $1 million announcement by the then Abbott government for it's 'Dob in a Dealer' hotline. On 26 May 2015, Nathan Barratt, a Northern Territory government MP and the chair of the Northern Territory government's inquiry into ice, flagged random, mandatory drug testing for private and public sectors, as well as for revellers on Darwin's nightclub strip.

According to the 2010 National Drug Strategy and Household Survey (NDSHS), a large majority of Australians — four out of five — supported tougher sentencing laws for the sale and supply of heroin, amphetamines, cocaine, and ecstasy. Similarly, a hypothetical distribution of $100 showed that a law-enforcement approach ($40.50) was favoured by Australians, as compared to the funds they would allocate for drug education ($33.80) and drug treatment ($25.70) in reducing illegal drug use.

There are few areas in public policy with such a significant gap between what the public wants and what the policy wonks and frontline workers think is best.

At the same time, expressing drug policy in Australia as a dichotomous and clear divide between a 'tough-on-drugs' approach and a 'harm minimisation' approach simply doesn't fit what has been, to date, a mixed-policy approach. The current regime, while undeniably and predominantly law-enforcement focused, has nonetheless become more progressive, evidence-based, and effective at reducing the extent and harms of drug abuse: particularly federally over the past thirty years.

Since 1985, Australia's drug policies have been guided by our National Drug Strategy (the NDS), which has three components: demand reduction, supply reduction, and harm minimisation. In the seventy years prior to that, an approach that prioritised law enforcement dominated our policy thinking. In fact, it was the murder of a prominent anti-cannabis campaigner, Donald Mackay, in 1977, combined with the emergence of the 'hippie era', and soldiers coming back from the Vietnam War with a significant amount of other drugs, that prompted several royal commissions, including the Australian Royal Commission of Inquiry into Drugs (the Williams Inquiry) in 1979. The federal inquiry, combined with similar state-level inquiries, all concluded we needed more laws, better laws, and more money for law enforcement. However, it also became clear that drug use and drug harms—including drug-related crime—were actually rising, along with the rise of HIV/AIDS, and policy-makers decided a new approach was needed.

This new approach brought with it some very new ideas: first, that drug use should be treated mainly as a health issue; and second, that drug use is a complex phenomenon that will never be entirely eliminated. While the majority of funds were still put into law enforcement, the approach was modified, and, importantly, the political authority for drug policy was moved from the federal Attorney-General's Department to the federal Department of Health.

Politicians are often quick to draw attention to or brand their approaches as 'tough' when they have strong elements of harm reduction. Indeed, there is evidence that the approach to drug policy at the highest levels is being increasingly — albeit incrementally and sometimes with 'two steps forward, one step back' — informed by research and what drug experts believe. Politicians will often lead their press statements and press releases with great detail on the 'tough' aspects of their policy plan, while new money for treatment is often buried; when the New South Wales Liberal government announced its lowering of the 'large commercial quantity' threshold in September 2015, buried toward the end of the announcement was the fact it had also spent $11 million on treatment.

Released in late 2015, a report from the Australian Strategic Policy Institute (ASPI) titled 'Methamphetamine: focusing Australia's national ice strategy on the problem, not the symptoms', suggested that the reduction of crystal-meth abuse in Canada served as an ongoing example of why treatment and education are better than policing (co-author Vernn White is a former police officer from Canada). At the same time, it noted that Australia's political approaches were often tougher in words than action. It cites, for instance, the 1997 Howard government's 'Tough on Drugs' strategy in response to the 1990s heroin surge. While the bulk of the 'Tough on Drugs' funding went to organisations such as the Australian Federal Police and the federal Customs Service (and in fact reprioritised funding to law enforcement), there was also funding for new treatment centres, upgrading of new treatment centres, and school education programs. The program also created a number of progressive new initiatives, such as the Illicit Drug Diversion Initiative to divert cannabis and other drug users out of the criminal justice system and into education/ treatment.

The United Nations Office on Drugs and Crime (UNODC) adds in their 2008 report 'Drugs Policy and Results in Australia' that, despite being called 'Tough on Drugs', the strategy also:

included proposals to enable the diversion of drug users from prison to treatment with a view to breaking the cycle of drug dependency and criminal behavior. In addition, the strategy also singled out the importance of research, notably towards prevention and treatment of illicit drug use, with a stronger focus on abstinence-based treatment and eventual re-integration of users into the community.

The UNODC report also argued that this was a successful policy mix noting that 'overall drug use increased 69% over the 1988–98 period, notably between 1995 and 1998' but also that 'between 1998 and 2007 overall illicit drug use declined close to 40%. Amphetamines use declined by 38%; cannabis use fell by close to 50%; and use of heroin dropped by an impressive 75%'.

These figures again remind us of just how much the arrival of crystal meth has rendered previous knowledge of drug treatment and drug policy at least partially redundant — not least of all, some argue, because despite this multi-faceted approach, there is still a heavy emphasis on law-enforcement spending.

In addition, governments have traditionally favoured mass-media advertising campaigns — for reasons that aren't all together clear. The biggest spend from the federal government before it announced its federal inquiry and ice taskforce (which I will talk about in the next chapter) was a $9 million mass-media advertising campaign that was launched 10 May 2015. The advert showed some of the worst consequences from crystal-meth addiction: psychosis; a woman in tears picking at her skin; a young man punching his mother in the face while his little sister looks on; a man head-butting a doctor in a hospital while two elderly patients watch; and a worker telling his boss he hasn't finished his work. Beyond showing dramatic events, the advert doesn't contain very much information at all about crystal meth. It is almost identical to a federal government anti-ice advert that ran in 2007, but with different actors.

There is evidence that in some cases TV drug adverts can have the opposite effect than intended: in *Drugs and Drugs Policy*, Kleiman, Caulkins, and Hawken say that 'even the best prevention programs have only modest effects', and studies have shown that the main reason for this is that youth are also exposed to 'thousands of hours of other social influences: friends, television, music, and other media'. Information-only prevention programs were abandoned in the 1960s and 1970s because they were found to actually increase drug use among younger populations.

National Drug Research Institute director Steve Allsop, who has studied the general effectiveness of anti-drug advertising campaigns, told the Victorian inquiry that these 'messages do not sit well with an individual's own experience (for example implying that ecstasy use will often lead to death when in fact such occurrences are rare) [and thus] may not be credible with the target audience, and have the potential to undermine confidence in other messages or strategies.' He adds that mass-media campaigns that strongly highlight the adverse impact of drug use may contribute to the stigmatisation and marginalisation of drug users 'thereby reducing the possibility that they will seek or be offered assistance'.

It would be difficult to accuse Australian governments of not reaching out to communities and experts for guidance on the best way to deal with crystal meth. As we know, crystal-meth use in Australia first surged in Victoria; about two years into the surge, the then Napthine government announced a parliamentary inquiry into crystal meth. The report for the Victorian parliamentary inquiry into crystal meth was tabled on 3 September 2014, making 54 recommendations based on 15 underlying principles. This 856-page report is one of the most extensive, well-balanced, evidence-based, and well thought-out research inquiries I have ever read. It remains one of the most comprehensive documents about crystal-meth policy publicly available all over the world. The report's recommendations were a mix of drug prevention plans, ideas for awareness campaigns, calls for specialist crystal-meth treatment programs, calls for more drug treatment centres, particularly in rural Victoria, specific plans for crackdown on precursors and organised crime, and an expansion of alternative justice programs such as drug courts.

The report also highlighted the way New Zealand reduced its methamphetamine problem with a specific methamphetamine plan. While New Zealand's problems weren't with crystal meth but with highly potent powdered methamphetamine pills, the associated issues gave the nation a similar shock to the one Australia experienced later with crystal meth. New Zealand had an even bigger meth problem than Australia did a decade ago, and thanks partially to some decisive government action, meth use in the general population has now dropped from 3 per cent to 0.9 per cent. So how did they do it? Well, in 2009, the New Zealand government developed its 'Methamphetamine Action Plan'.

The package had five essential elements:

1. Crack down on precursors.
2. Break supply chains.
3. Provide better routes into treatment.
4. Support communities.
5. Strengthen governance.

Speaking to ABC Radio Central Victoria, Ross Bell, executive director of the New Zealand Drug Foundation, said:

> We got the initial response wrong; we thought a traditional law and enforcement approach worked. We thought we could just

stop the supply, but this didn't make any impact. Instead, we made an effort to decrease the stigma attached to meth users in the community ... and increased the number of people convicted of meth convictions going into drug treatment programs.

Bell explained that most of the new money going in to the program was invested in treatment, and making sure that more treatment beds were available, as a way of ensuring that if somebody needed help, it could be given to them.

Then, in May 2015, Victoria became the first Australian state to develop its own methamphetamine action plan: the 'Ice Action Plan'. Like New Zealand's and Canada's plans before it, it focused on a combination of harm reduction, reduced access to the drug, and increased services and treatment options. It also identified a need for building 'workforce capacity' by focusing on the violence experienced by frontline workers, and by structuring specific training and support for those workers.

The Andrews government later announced a $45.5 million spend to implement the plan—$18 million would be used 'to expand drug treatment and rehabilitation' for ice users. A further $15 million was allocated to new drug-and-booze buses, $4.5 million to expand Victoria police forensic teams to crack down on clandestine drug labs, and $4.7 million to help support ice users and their families, including a new ice helpline.

For many, there are clear positives in the plan, as it indicates a shift in funding proportion from law enforcement to information and treatment. A $45 million increase in drug-treatment services is nothing to be sneezed at. The Andrews government said this funding would create about 500 new residential rehab beds each year not to mention other new drug treatment services in areas, like Pakenham, where the population's growth has moved significantly faster than its infrastructure. So for instance, in Narre Warren — a central suburb in the Victoria City of Casey (near Pakenham) that now has a bigger population than Canberra — there is now funding to run a new specialist drug program that will provide rehabilitation services in an area that previously had almost none.

However, a question many are left with is: why wasn't there *more* money spent on treatment services? If we compare this plan to the successful New Zealand plan, it is clear the approaches are very similar; it is also clear, though, that unlike the New Zealand model, there is no standalone provision for more places in treatment 'for problematic methamphetamine users' or for better routes into treatment.

One key set of recommendations from the Victorian report was ignored in the subsequent Ice Action Plan. The parliamentary committee recommended the expansion of the Drug Court of Victoria. Commencing in May 2002, the court currently operates in just one location — Dandenong — and diverts drug dependent offenders into treatment.

Three years after the court started, Turning Point Alcohol and Drug Centre and Health Outcomes International carried out a joint evaluation, which found: a drug-court program graduation rate of 15 per cent with a projected completion rate of 30 per cent per annum in subsequent years once the program had become more established; a reduction in unemployment rates of participants by 32 per cent; significant reductions in re-offending rates (graduates re-offended 68 per cent less than a 'control group' of non-drug-court criminal offenders) — leading the researchers to conclude that for every $1 the program uses, the community dividend is $5.

Australian drug courts were largely based on models that were developed in the United States. Under Californian law introduced in 2000, 35,000 people convicted of drug or drug-related offences have been diverted from jail to drug treatment — half of these people were methamphetamine addicts. Ethan Nadelmann, executive director of the US-Based Drug Policy Alliance testified before Congress in 2010: 'A recent evaluation by the University of California Los Angeles (UCLA) found that California taxpayers saved nearly $2.50 for every dollar invested in the program. Of people who successfully completed their drug treatment, California taxpayers saved nearly $4 for each dollar spent. In all, Proposition 36 is estimated to have saved state and local government more than $1.3 billion over its first six years.'

The Victorian parliamentary committee suggested expanding an alternative justice program that runs in Melbourne, Sunshine, and the Latrobe Valley, but that recommendation was also ignored.

If we widen our lens a little more, it is clear just how much state and territory governments' love for 'law-and-order' may be limiting the amount of money it could spend on all types of health and education services—including those that relate to crystal-meth abuse. The Andrews government will spend $18 million on crystal-meth treatment; its budget that year set aside $243 million for upgrading and expanding prisons, and another $90 million for the Department of Corrections to assist them in administering community corrections orders. In delivering its 2015–16 budget, the New South Wales government dedicated $11 million to better drug rehabilitation services; at the same time, it dedicated nearly $7 billion of its $70 billion state budget to 'public order and safety' (keeping it in line with Victoria and Queensland state governments who also spend about 10 per cent of their budgets on 'public order and safety'), announcing that the government would 'appoint 310 new police officers by 2018, including 250 specialist police and 15 specialist civilian staff'. By the end of 2018, police numbers are expected to reach 16,795, up from 15,806 in 2011 when the government came to power.

In 1982, there were 9,826 Australians in prison. In 2015,

there were 36,134. I looked across different Australian Bureau of Statistics (ABS) data from the last three decades, and found that the per capita rate of imprisonment has doubled since I was born in 1980: from 92 per 100,000 people in 1982 to 186 prisoners per 100,000 in 2015 (a rise again from 158 per 100,000 in 2004). Our prison system is funded and administered by state and territory governments, and people are imprisoned as a result of state and territory law. Crimes against the person such as assault account for the biggest rise, followed by drug offences: just over 3,000 of Australia's prisoners are in there for drug offences—which is a 10-fold growth increase since 1982.

If you are charged with a drug offence in Australia you will either be charged with possession (having two grams or less for most drugs, including methamphetamine—two years in prison is the maximum penalty), or trafficking. The ACC's 2014–15 Illicit Drug Data report reveals 79,070 people were charged with drug offences during that period, and 66 per cent, or just over 52,000, of them were charged with possession. Over the same period, 112,049 people were arrested for suspected drug offences (evidently not everyone arrested is charged, and not everyone charged with drug offences goes to court, instead receiving fines); 59 per cent of those were arrested for cannabis charges, and 87 per cent of those arrests are for possession-only charges.

As remarkable as this may appear, it's not the most remarkable fact about drug offences in Australia: that title almost certainly belongs to a statistic I found in a relatively obscure section of an ABS data series called 'Finalised Defendants', which measures the number of people going to court as defendants and the types of offences they had been charged with. The data shows that the number one offence an Australian will be charged with and required to go to court for is a drug offence. In 2013–14, there were 579,152 cases completed in Australia's criminal courts: 10 per cent of them were for drug offences, and of those roughly

50,000 cases, 28,000 were there for drug possession. To express this in another way: about 5 per cent of everybody in Australia who goes to court does so because they were caught with less than two grams of drugs. The overall trend of drug offences, and in particular drug possession offences, is up and up: the number of defendants finalised with a principal offence of illicit drug offences increased by 15 per cent or 6,442 defendants.

Alison Ritter's 2011 study showed that the biggest sub-group within drug-related law-enforcement costs was police services and correctional services work, which shows why, in essence, most of the money directed at drug-policy law enforcement has been spent on the costs of employing and administering police officers. When we consider this in the context of the ACC's Drug Data Report and the ABS Finalised Defendants scheme, what the study demonstrates is that about $700 million a year — twice the amount of the total state, territory, and federal government spend on drug treatment — was being spent on police activities and correctional services related to charging, arresting, and prosecuting people for possessing an amount of illicit drugs — usually marijuana — deemed by the law itself to be for personal use only. At the same time, addicts and frontline workers continue to cite a lack of treatment services as the biggest barrier to reducing personal and social harms arising from drug abuse.

By way of example — and it is quite an acute example of drug-related expenditure on law and order — let me take you to Queensland, which has the highest number of illicit drug arrests in the nation. Arrests for cannabis use and possession are particularly high: nearly five times more people are arrested for cannabis use here than in more populated Victoria. Between 2010 and 2015, the number of people behind bars in Queensland has increased by more than 20 per cent. As a result, nine of the state's 11 high-security prisons are now filled beyond capacity, resulting in an increase in staff and inter-prisoner assaults. When the Queensland Newman government came to power in 2012, it promised to balance the budget and get tough on crime. This meant less money for specialist courts, legal aid, and youth social programs, and more money for the police. Newman's Liberal National Party government axed the Murri Court, the Drug Court (which had been operating in Beenleigh, Ipswich, Southport, Cairns, and Townsville) and the Special Circumstances Courts (for those offenders with mental-health issues). It also wound back several prison work programs. The Newman government then funded 1,100 extra police, at a cost of $358 million (though when the Australian Labor Party Palaszczuk government was elected in 2015, it quietly restored the Murri Court, the Drug Court, and the Special Circumstances Courts).

Now Queensland Crime Stoppers is funded by the state government. As you no doubt already know, it is designed so people can call in and report crime anonymously. This information is handed over to the police. I stumbled across a press release from the organisation from February 2016 boasting that: 'Reports made to Crime Stoppers Queensland in 2015 led to 2,622 arrests and 9,452 charges being placed, which is a significant increase'.

However, 9,105 of those 9,452 charges related to drug possession and supply. A further 36 were for drug trafficking. Which left just a few other offences to make up the other 300 or so charges: five child pornography offences, 12 prostitution offences, 31 breaches of bail offences, two rape offences (but no murders or assaults).

'These are the best statistics we've seen since our program commenced in 1989, and it's the third consecutive year our program has broken historical records for the number of arrests resulting from community information reports,' the press release continued.

History is crucial to understanding how and why Australian states and territories ended up spending so much of their money on arresting, charging, and attempting to prosecute people for using certain mind-altering substance.

Australia's legislative position has, in effect, come from several major international treaties. In the early twentieth century, opium use in China was considered to be very detrimental to the local population, and British traders were exploiting the local Chinese population through the opium trade. The British government removed their support for the opium trade, and a short time later the Chinese government banned opium altogether. A few years later, the International Opium Commission was founded and an International Opium Convention was signed by 13 nations at The Hague in 1912. This amounted to the world's first drug control treaty, and would be later registered at the League of Nations in 1922. Effectively it meant that all signatory nations to the treaty, which later became part of the much larger Treaty of Versailles, had made the sale, distribution, and use of narcotic drugs illegal, unless they were used for medical or scientific purposes. This convention was revised again in 1925. In 1961, the Narcotics Convention made this a binding contract, as members signed an agreement that they would keep the use of certain plants and substances illegal. Following that was the 1971 Convention on Psychotropic Substances — a United Nations treaty designed to cover a range of new psychoactive drugs not covered in the 1961 convention. This included methamphetamine, which was all but completely outlawed in Australia by 1976. So it was ultimately the interpretation and application of these conventions by member-states including Australia that led to drug use, not just drug supply, being made illegal all around the western world.

And for some, criminalisation of drug use is at the core of why drug harms continue to occur across our societies. In July 2001, the Portuguese government decriminalised the use, possession, and acquisition of all illicit drugs, including cannabis, heroin, amphetamines, and ecstasy, when deemed for personal use. However, it is still illegal for a person to possess illicit drugs, and if a person is found by police to have illicit drugs they are referred to a special panel comprised of a treatment professional, a social worker, and a lawyer. All other drug offences, including trafficking-consumption, trafficking, manufacturing, and cultivation continue to be criminal offences with punishment of up to twelve years' imprisonment.

The results have been reported as both a success and as a failure by different sides of the argument, but what is clear is that although there was a slight increase in the use of all illicit drugs in the general population between 2001 and 2007, the levels of 'problematic drug use, HIV, and offending' all saw a reduction. The biggest change was in the drop in drug-related new HIV infections: these decreased between 2000 and 2009 from 1,400 to fewer than 200 cases per year.

Other countries in Latin America have followed the same path, but it is too early to measure the effectiveness of drug decriminalisation in countries such as Venezuela, Colombia, and Uruguay.

For me, the three strongest arguments in favour of decriminalising crystal meth, or any drug for that matter, are these: first, the proposed decriminalisation and legalisation is about the use of small quantities, meaning drug traffickers would still face jail time. Second, the idea really centres around good use of resources—money that would usually be spent on arresting, prosecuting, and convicting individual users could be spent instead on chasing higher-end dealers and investing in better treatment services. And third, although it is difficult to imagine a world in which substances such as methamphetamine, cocaine, and heroin are legal, drug prohibition is very much grounded in recent history.

And for many around the world, the 'prohibitionist approach' to narcotic and amphetamine use is just not working. The Global Commission on Drug Policy, a 22-person panel that issued an assessment in 2011 of the global 'War on Drugs', opened its report with the following sentence:

> The global war on drugs has failed, with devastating consequences for individuals and societies around the world.

The commission is headed by the former secretary-general of the United Nations, Kofi Annan, a number of former presidents and prime ministers (including those of Brazil, Colombia, Greece, Portugal, Switzerland, and Chile), businessmen, intellectuals, and senior administrators from around the world. The commission called for a reopening of the debate on drugs policy, and recommended that regulation ultimately replace prohibition. Speaking at a World Economic Forum in Switzerland in 2013, Annan said 'I believe that drugs have destroyed many people, but wrong governmental policies have destroyed many more … When we realised [alcohol] prohibition wasn't working we had the courage to change it.' Based on the data outlined in this chapter, I believe there is a convincing argument to be made that too many resources are being spent arresting and prosecuting individual users when the money could be better spent elsewhere.

I asked the researcher Nicole Lee, whose work I have quoted earlier in this book, what she thought of, respectively, decriminalisation and legalisation of meth. Lee told me that in general, she is in favour of decriminalisation of all illicit drugs:

> Criminalisation is based on a conservative moral view about drugs and has been, globally, heavily driven by prohibitionist countries like the US and others (e.g. Sweden) for many decades. It increases harms and stigma and reduces our ability to provide treatment to those who need it. Treatment is more efficient and

cost effective in reducing drug use and harms than policing. I think in Australia the couple of states that decriminalised cannabis show that it doesn't increase drug use or problems. And the Portuguese experience, a fairly bold move, shows more benefits than harms. Legalisation is a different, more complex issue, but I think decriminalisation is a good step to reducing harms among drug users and for the community.

Other supporters of decriminalisation include former Australian Federal Police commissioner Mick Palmer, former New South Wales premier Bob Carr, and ASPI's Vern White. The 'Geelong Our Town's ICE Fight' lead project officer Police Senior Sergeant Tony Francis has also called for decriminalisation. The *Geelong Advertiser* published his comments, along with a response from Premier Andrews, who has ruled out the possibility of decriminalising ice, as has Nationals senator Fiona Nash, who is both the assistant minister for health and the government head of the National Ice Taskforce that was launched on 7 April 2015.

Nash was actually quoted from a press release in which she plainly conflated legalisation and decriminalisation: 'However, legalising the drug would send the message that ice is not dangerous. This is the wrong message to send. Legalising what is arguably the worst drug Australia has seen is madness.'

But it is again important to point out the nuance in this debate — Nash can hardly be characterised as a hard-liner, also saying: 'During my recent 25,000-kilometre tour holding community consultations on ice — I've now done so in 12 regional communities — police of all ranks have repeatedly told me we can't arrest our way out of the ice problem. I've been open to new suggestions and understand a range of measures is needed. Education is key — we must teach our young people about the dangers of ice. There's no need to exaggerate the message — the truth is scary enough.'

Perhaps even more telling was that the then Abbott government appointed Ken Lay, former Victorian police commissioner, to the role of taskforce head. Lay's most famous remark about Australia's ice problem had been up to that point that 'we can't arrest our way out of the ice problem'.

A Fairfax/Nielsen poll taken in 2012 found that two-thirds of Australians oppose decriminalisation. The poll showed 27 per cent of voters support decriminalisation, although that figure rose to 50 per cent of Greens and 34 per cent of Labor voters. Support among Liberal and National party voters was much lower, at 18 per cent. The poll results were almost exactly the same as they were when taken thirteen years earlier. Attitudes seem pretty fixed — just 4 per cent of respondents said they neither supported nor opposed decriminalisation, and 2 per cent said they did not know.

In any event, Australia will be unlikely to make any serious changes to criminalisation until there is a change in some of these international treaties, and for that to happen, it would need America's support.

Another side of the debate, and one that is similarly about the role of government, is the extent to which the harms associated with the crystal-meth surge are only symptomatic of other service gaps and social problems. The author James Fry, whose memoir *That Fry Boy* was released in early 2015, published an article in September 2015 in which he identified underfunding as the main problem facing people seeking access to appropriate drug and alcohol support:

> Critics against the allocation of scarce public funds towards mental health are right to say that to bring the system up to an effective level, one that could rapidly respond to the Janes of the world when they need it most, would be very costly. But such critics fail to acknowledge that when we are not providing

rapid access to mental-health treatment we default to providing
far more costly responses to the problem. Largely this takes the
form of law enforcement and emergency departments.

Fry's comments are important because they suggest that gaps
in mental-health services are now joining up with gaps in drug
and alcohol treatment, and, I would further suggest, with gaps in
a lack of affordable housing to create ever-growing gaping holes.

It is, perhaps, worth reflecting here on the issue of ideology
and the role of government. Since the 1980s, and under
neoliberalism, the government's role has been, in theory at least,
to help people help themselves, determined that it would not
be seen as a panacea for all social ills. In another paper from
2011, 'An assessment of illicit drug policy in Australia', Alison
Ritter explored the move in the 1980s from governments
'rowing' to 'steering', suggesting that it has particularly impacted
on drug policy and service provision. These changes in the
provision of services, traditionally government-run and now
privatised (including not-for-profits within this definition),
are consistent with pluralised governance. Known by various
terms — harnessing of non-state resources; co-production; multi-
lateralisation; interagency/multi-agency partnerships; third-party
policing; and hybrid governance — this new mentality reflects
an acknowledgement that the state has limited resources, cannot
manage everything in the best way, and that non-state actors can
play an effective role.

Australia's crystal-meth surge occurred after the GFC, and
while we came out of that largely unscathed, it did have an impact
on unemployment, which rose from 4 per cent previously to
6 per cent by the start of 2010, and has since hovered somewhere
between 5 per cent and 6.5 per cent. Since 2011, job vacancies
have dropped around 25 per cent. Youth unemployment has been
particularly high: in 2015, the official unemployment rate for

15–24-year-olds was, at 14 per cent, the highest since 1998. The Australian Institute of Health and Welfare's 2015 report showed that in 2013, 24.9 per cent of unemployed people reported that they had used illicit drugs in the past twelve months, compared with 16.8 per cent of employed people.

Former Victorian premier Jeff Kennett has said that one of the major reasons for the increasing prevalence of ice addiction is the growth in youth unemployment: 'We don't have any idea of how we are going to grow society in a way that will provide employment for those who are out of work—and that's a failing of the political system on both sides,' he told *The Sydney Morning Herald* in April 2015.

Geoff Munro from the Australian Drug Foundation told me he thinks that the cyclical nature of drug taking means that even if methamphetamine were taken out of the picture, a new and potentially more harmful drug may be abused in its place:

I think we have had a bit of a breakdown in our community and we need to re-think the way we operate. We need to create a better framework for our children, we need to re-engage the extended family in children's lives, we need to make sure children have a wider network who taken an interest in them. We need to make sure schools are creating a better environment, we need to make sure we are building a society that overcomes social disadvantage and that is helping people build a kind of emotional framework that is strong and deep enough so they don't feel the need to abuse drugs. We need better early intervention for mental health, we need actual psychologists in public schools, and we need to make sure schools are helping us build a cohesive society, were people feel like they have a place. Unless we look at what kind of society we are creating then all these other ways of treating problem drug users are merely a band-aid.

## Chapter Sixteen

# Beyond excess

STU FENTON, FORTY-TWO, is ruggedly handsome and softly spoken. Ten years ago, he found that despite joining Narcotics Anonymous, and despite trying to take on what he was being taught, he was still going on crystal-meth binges. Nearly every time he did, he had recurring psychotic delusions: his prior sexual encounters were being shown on a television channel or being broadcast somewhere in a public space. It was either that, or he believed that the police were going to arrest and imprison him for something, or perhaps for nothing in particular — just for being himself.

Fenton told me that there was no apparent reason for when he called it quits other than he was exhausted. He moved into a residential rehab. He stayed for ten months. During that time, he thought through his early childhood on a rural Victorian farm, and, when searching his mind after I asked him for an example, he ummed and ahhed before finally saying: 'It might sound trivial, but my dad never picked me up, never hugged me, never told he loved me.' Fenton grew up in his small country town to find other boys didn't like him because he was gay; this was during the 1980s, and at the height of the AIDS epidemic.

During his time in rehab, he began to feel a deep shame that he related back to his sexuality, and this shame played out in the delusion that his sex life was being played on televisions for all to see. These emotional realisations were only a starting point, though: 'I think when I developed a belief in a higher power, that really finally allowed me to move on from drug abuse and drug addiction,' Fenton told me. 'I am not talking about God, but something greater than yourself. Once I found that greater power then I started praying to it; it was like a life force, a higher intelligence, and it gave me a great sense of energy. It made me want to live life for the here and now.'

Over time he said he became 'other-centred' instead of self-seeking. Today, nearly ten years clean, he said part of the process has been abstaining from *all* things—he hasn't had a drink of alcohol or smoked a cigarette since.

Jack Nagle (who you may remember as the guy who thought he was living in a 'Truman Show' world) told me that he quit crystal meth shortly after that 10-day binge during which he smoked $7,500 worth of the drug. 'It was standing in front of the mirror that I had a moment of clarity. It sounds funny to say, but the truth just kind of dawned on me—I stopped worrying about being filmed or being followed, and I just saw myself for what I was. I had dropped down to 66 kilos and for someone who is nearly 200 centimetres tall, that is bone-thin.'

After going through rehab, he, too, came to see his delusions of being recorded as having their roots in a deep sense of shame. 'I think I was just quite insecure about myself … I always thought of myself as not being smart enough.'

Cassy McDonald sent me a Facebook message: 'I did manage to get clean on my own without seeing a counsellor, but I found that when I quit I had a "feel for the steel" so I was shooting up water with syringe even after I stopped using just because I liked the routine of using it.'

In *Memoirs of an Addicted Brain* neuroscientist and former coke- and meth-addict Marc Lewis talks about a two-year period after a lifetime of drug use where his life was a 'wide-open passage to nowhere'.

He described this time as consisting of periods of 'resolve, even peacefulness, interspersed by bouts of depression'. Eventually, Lewis starting working at a crisis centre for street kids; he became a development psychologist, and then a professor, before taking up his main gig in emotional neuroscience.

'You could say my life became too full even to consider a return to drugs but that wouldn't tell the full story. Not all the sculpting of synapses in my early twenties is irrevocable. The meaning of drugs, the imagined value they represent, is still inscribed in my orbito-frontal cortex ... As is well known in addiction lore there is no final cure, just recovery, abstention and self-awareness. But there *are* happy endings.'

I found it tempting to write a joke here about how there are definitely 'happy endings' to be found in crystal meth, particularly when one masturbates. More so, though, I was loath to write a 'happy ending' when drug addiction more generally, and this book more specifically, deals with so many stories that end with anything but a meaningful resolution.

Writing an ending with a resolution is deeply problematic, too, when you consider the trajectory of Smithy and Beck. By the time I got to Melbourne, I was afraid to ask the few people I knew who had stayed in contact with them how they fared—particularly after they lost custody of the twins (and I was very conscious of my part in that).

And back in Melbourne, admittedly, I was often too deep in delusion or too distracted by simply surviving, to fully consider the fate of my former friends. Even the most terrible habits can be comfortable and comforting, and so, with no further ado, let me tell you about my crystal-meth relapse, which started in a half-empty, two-bedroom brick unit in Noble Park in early 2015. A relapse that must have occurred, let's see, about a week after I got back to Melbourne from Bundaberg. In truth — just as when I had left rehab in 2008 — I hadn't made a commitment to go 100 per cent clean. Despite seeing the obvious danger in using again, I had cravings for the drug, even on the plane (or especially on the plane because of the way it mimics *that* feeling) that made me daydream, shift excitedly on my seat, and begin to drool.

The night I relapsed I didn't actually seek it out, but drugs aren't hard to find when most of your friends are people you met through drugs or clubs. A guy named Steven whom I had met in a nightclub about a decade prior contacted me via Facebook: he was moving out of his house, and asked if I wanted to come over and 'hang out in the garage'. When I got there, I found that he was off his dial on crystal meth, and we soon ordered more. I smoked it and smoked it and smoked it all night with him in that musty, cluttered garage — sitting on an esky, on a cool summer night, as we plummeted the pleasurable 'depths' of our bullshit and shallow self-love. In fact, it is fair to say I smoked until I went cross-eyed, and until I got out a piece of paper and started writing. I did some work on a creative writing piece, and for some reason during this, I started thinking about a bad argument I'd had with one of Steven's friends many moons earlier. I began to think that he had only invited me over to make fun of me, and that what we'd smoked wasn't really crystal meth. Then everything Steven said began to be interpreted through this psychotic prism — my ideas were resistant to whatever he said, so resistant that everything he said simply reinforced the idea that he was up to something really quite sinister. So even when he broke into his own psychosis, and believed that police had surrounded the house (Steven has never got into trouble with the law), I thought that this, too, was part of his nasty plot against me.

Eventually, I left, and caught an early morning train. I thought that everyone on the train was talking about me and staring at me—words people said were references to me, and any look in my direction made me feel as if they knew everything that was bad about me. I had begun to wonder how people knew all this, and I concluded that the Coffee Club incident had been broadcast around Melbourne. It felt as if the interior of Melbourne's bright-green and yellow modern trains had served up some kind of proverbial hell where I was being judged and punished for all my sins. When I got to the city, I got off and caught the tram, and again I couldn't look anybody in the eye because I felt so guilty and so ashamed.

I went to the Alfred; I wanted to be in a locked psych ward because I was worried that with this level of public humiliation I would eventually crack and kill myself. At the counter, I saw a nurse who spoke in a stern Irish tone, and the first thing I did was apologise to her. I told her I was sorry to all the women at the hospital for everything that I had done, and that I knew that I was on the news.

'I'm a mess of different things that don't all go together,' I told her.

I was admitted straightaway. I told the next nurse I saw about how I was worried I was on the news.

'Oh, honey,' she said with a warm smile. 'You are not on the news; I'll go and speak to a doctor.' She came back with a small yellow pill, and said, 'Put this under your tongue until it dissolves, and if you feel like lying down after that you are more than welcome.' After a very short period of time, perhaps less than ten minutes, I felt very, very tired. So I rested in the small white room, with the door open, until it hit me—'I've been psychotic'—and I left with my tail between my legs.

So while it was fair to say I was nonplussed by life in general, it was after this incident that I began to form a new conclusion:

Crystal meth was just as predictable as everything else in my life.

Thereafter, I tried living ordinary waking life to its fullest in Melbourne. I didn't have any work at that time, but I exercised, I went for walks, I read a lot, I sought to be as kind and open to everyone as possible. One day I went to the cinema, I went out for dinner, I went out to the gym, I read, I walked around Melbourne. It was pleasant, and I felt good, very good, but I was left with two complementary emotions: 'this still isn't enough, I want more' and 'that was a nice day; wouldn't it be even nicer to finish it off with some crystal meth?'

Later that day, I met up with an old school friend.

We had used together in the past, and I knew we would use again that night. We got drunk, and eventually I suggested we get some crystal meth—this time, I got a syringe and injected it. I did not go into psychosis, but it was the same old Fantasia, in which we exchanged tales about how good and how underappreciated we were. After that I went back to The Gatwick, the notorious St Kilda hotel I was staying in to research an article, and masturbated for twelve hours—alone, stuck in the same repetitive, amoral sexual fantasies that I would never carry out in real life. It was boring, and I wondered if I could ever get my addiction under control. I went to a St Kilda drug clinic, where I was told it would take four days to see a GP and ten days to see a drug counsellor. Over the next two weeks:

I read Viktor Frankl's *Man's Search for Meaning*.

I read Mihaly Csikszentmihalyi's *Flow: the psychology of optimal experience*.

I daydreamed about my trip to Asia.

I started drinking most nights in St Kilda's Fitzroy Street bars.

I came back to the musty, grotty Gatwick one night drunk, and saw a woman injecting crystal meth in her neck. When I asked her why she was injecting it in her neck she said, 'Straight to the brain, brother'.

She huffed and puffed, eyes wild, before introducing me to the woman standing behind her: her daughter, Anna, who repeated her mother's ritual with her own syringe. 'Are you sure you don't want some, love?' she asked, and I answered yes, of course I did.

Anna took me to a room—let's say room number 666—where I was handed a point of meth for $100, and a clean syringe still in its packet, and I went back to the bathroom and injected the old-fashioned way—on the inside of my elbow.

Over the course of the night, I bought and injected some more with a young homeless man with autism, who spent the entire time we were injecting reciting tracts from what seemed to be a high school science book off the top of his head.

My bank account ran dry.

I forgot my bank account ran dry.

I ordered more meth off a guy I remember as The Bald Man and his dodgy-looking goons.

He followed me to the ATM.

When he realised my bank account was empty, he went ballistic, threatening me, and ripping the chains from my neck, and telling me I could expect to be visited by him later and have my jaw broken.

I retreated to my Gatwick room, where I saw maggots crawling all over the floor, and a series of detailed plots began to form in my head. As the morning progressed, I concluded that somebody had broken into my room while I was out and had stolen my laptop to give to a journalist who had hijacked my internet history—my internet porn history, to be precise—and broadcast it on the news.

In no time, it was a bright late-summer morning.

It dawned on me that I couldn't ask my parents for money.

I went to the St Kilda Crisis Centre. While waiting outside, a woman came up to me, with the regular two eyes most humans have, and told me one of her eyes had been stolen.

I believed she was part of the mob who were after me, and that she was telling me my eyes would be cut out. And on it went. I visited my publisher during this time as well, believing that they wanted to cancel the book. I tried to access crisis housing, but was told it was full.

Eventually, I had to return to the Gatwick.

During my sessions with Jay in Bundaberg, she told me many things, and two in particular stuck in my mind while I was at the Gatwick: the first was to think about drug addiction like 'a stray cat that you don't want to feed; the more you feed it the more it keeps coming back', and the second was that I needed to take responsibility.

By the end of my third relapse, I decided, that yes, I was very much over crystal meth. But there was still the pressing question of what freedom from drugs and freedom from addiction would mean for me, and indeed, what freedom means for me more generally.

In *Being and Nothingness,* Jean Paul Sartre writes: 'We do not know what we want and yet we are responsible for what we are—that is the fact.' While I can admit that Sartre—albeit just my first-year philosophy understanding of him—wasn't on my mind when I was at the Gatwick, freedom, responsibility, and their respective limits were. The Gatwick was a place full of people whose notions of freedom and responsibility are surely limited by both madness and economics. The extent to which Australia's underclass are trapped in their existence occurred to me shortly after my final binge at the Gatwick. Yet many of its inhabitants remained joyous at times; self-pity was kept to a minimum, and people were doing their best to find meaning in the abject and grossly unfair economic conditions that most of them couldn't escape.

I don't quote Sartre's work here to justify a kind of 'cult of the will' — it is about people's capacity to make their own meaning of their situation. Sartre would in later life become a militant neo-Marxist who saw economic scarcity as an obvious limit on human freedom — the point being that one cannot be free or authentic when all your energy is expended on finding the next meal or on feeding your family.

The Gatwick taught me first and foremost about the dire state of housing in Australia (there are 34,000 people on the public-housing waiting list in Victoria alone), and the people there showed me that my experiences of the world didn't justify me seeing things in such a dim way. I wasn't entitled to take drugs because of my suffering. My drug use felt childish and decadent — I was surrendering my obligation to make meaning out of an often-absurd world to a drug that I knew would make me psychotic.

After my third relapse, I decided to stop using for the remainder of my time in Melbourne, and eventually I caught a plane to Malaysia.

I travelled from Kuala Lumpur to Penang to Phuket, and then to a sizzling hot, cat-piss stained, communal-living 'art space' on the fringes of Bangkok city. Curious, short on cash, I shared a room with ten other people that was covered in paintings and graffiti and poetry, and cost just over $4 a night.

I had arrived, in my ignorance, just in time for Bangkok's hot, humid April. It was 37 degrees every day with 80 per cent humidity; the art-space was in a five-storey building in a non-tourist part of town, and it was permanently boiling inside it.

I must have been there no more than a week when I had a fight with a young English guy that started me on a new train of thought: *why am I so angry? Why am I the only person unable to cope with the sweltering conditions?*

In the cold — make that obscenely hot and sweaty — light of day, I began to think that I was a very angry man. My anger was making me unhappy, I was having trouble escaping it, and it was making a very nasty, unpleasant person at times. I wondered if it was the after-effects of crystal meth? A part of my personality that grew and grew during months of drug use, and had then become part of who I was? I knew, though, that in truth I had been full of rage for a long time.

Prior to this time, I had never read about anger — at least not from a personal perspective. I had always been focused on the things that made me angry, deciding that I would rather be angry than passive, and that there were things worth fighting for and getting angry about.

About an hour's walk away from the art-space was Khao San Road, the tourist area of Bangkok, renowned for its trashiness and its often trashy book stands. Walking past one day, I spotted *Buddha* by one of my favourite authors: the ex-nun Karen Armstrong. I read her biography of the Gautama, *Buddha*, as well as *Siddhartha* by Hermann Hesse. The story of the Buddha was so simple, and it started to make a lot of sense to me.

Guatama was born into a rich family, perhaps a royal family. When he first left his family, he saw many people suffering from physical pain, poverty, and also from old age. He went to try to discover why so many people suffered. At first he starved himself, inflicted himself with pain, and sought what we might call 'altered states of consciousness'. This nearly killed him. He decided he needed to find a balance between nihilism and self-indulgence, so he spent many years meditating in the jungle, and discovered what we today call 'Enlightenment' — an experience that is beyond the power of words to describe.

Buddhism involves a complex number of teachings and ideas, but the starting point resonated with me — namely that the cause of human suffering, or *dukkha*, is desire, and that the alternative to desire is enlightenment. I wanted to be on the path to enlightenment.

The Wat Phra That Doi Suthep (aka The Golden Temple) sits halfway up a Himalayan mountain directly facing Chiang Mai city in Northern Thailand. It's a half-hour tuk-tuk drive up the Doi Suthep mountain to reach the temple. The mountain landscape changes about every three or four kilometres along the incline: from dry bamboo forest to wet, mossy landscapes to flowers, to mixtures of all three. Until finally you arrive at the temple, with its 20-foot Buddha at the entrance of 230 steps, surrounded by jungle park, with cool misty air that smells of the forest surrounding it, and views over Chiang Mai—the city of one million emerging as just one valley among endless Himalayan rises.

At the temple, I saw a sign for the 'Vipassana Mindfulness Silent Meditation Centre'. Vipassana means 'to see things as they really are'. I had tried mindfulness in Australia in a silly psychology clinic about three years earlier and found it completely unhelpful. In fact, I regarded the application of mindfulness in the West as nothing but another fad in the discipline of psychology—which, to date, had been hit-and-miss in providing me with the help I often felt I needed. But there was something about the Golden Temple that made me feel that it was worth trying. I went in to make an inquiry, and was told I needed to make a booking, and that the course was by donation only.

I spent a few more weeks in Chiang Mai, staying in a hostel, abstaining from everything. I found a new level of hunger for the company of others as well as for reading, including some of the 'difficult novels' and a book called *Wisdom of the Buddha: the unabridged Dhammapada*.

This was all well and good, until I ran out of money again. I emailed the vipassana centre, and they said I could pay just $2 a day if I wanted, but I had to follow a number of ethical precepts as well as the 'Terms of Abstaining', which included abstaining from stealing, 'false speech' (actually, we weren't allowed to talk at all), singing, dancing, eating after noon, and over-indulging in sleep.

A few days later, I enrolled and was shown the basic meditation technique. I participated in an introductory ceremony in a big hall with the head monk, Sunny. I sat in lotus position in front of him as he sat in his bright orange robes, and, as required, I had to sing a hymn in Thai, then present him with some flowers.

'You may think you are your name, your job, who your friends are, what you thinking, what you are thinking—but there is a deeper level to your Self and that is what you are here to find,' he told me.

And then there was nothing to do, no talking, no TV, no reading or writing—nothing to do except meditate.

Fourteen hours a day just sitting and breathing, slow-walking and meditating in front of Buddha statues. I was told to notice my thoughts, but to not attach to them—rather, I was to just watch them float away. While I believed I had already thought through my anger, all the thoughts I had were angry thoughts—anger with my parents, anger about triple j, anger about high school. There were no distractions, and it all felt so unpleasant. It made it nearly impossible for me to meditate.

I was looking forward to my meeting with Sunny; I hoped he would offer me some words of advice to help me with these awful feelings. When we sat down together the next day, he asked me how meditation was going, and I said, 'I feel so angry, I just keep—' and he cut right in: 'Yes, yes, yes,' he said. 'Everyone finds it difficult, what you need to do is just breathe.' And then he sang, 'Rising, falling, rising, falling, rising, falling.'

And then: 'I'll see you tonight for the evening chant.'

Apparently Buddhism is *not* psychotherapy. Words were cheap at the Doi Suthep. Western philosophy privileges thought; many strands of eastern philosophy do not.

I spent all the next day just breathing out slowly and not being able to concentrate, and getting hungrier and more fatigued, and exhausted. Then the evening chant—all of us sitting on the floor, chanting together for forty-five minutes.

And then prayer. I was still light-headed from the lack of food and sleep, but this somehow made me feel serene, almost trance-like, and I could start to focus on the stillness, a bit and then a bit more. An angry thought came up—this one about my parents—and I just kept breathing, and it seemed to fade away through lack of significance. And then after more chanting, and three solid minutes of meditation, I experienced for the first time moments of near-complete stillness and the thoughts stopped. When the angry thoughts came up again, I was flushed with visions of red and purple and pink as the images dissipated and broke down. These colours became spectacular tropical flowers that danced around in my head, and suddenly I had deep feelings of awe and calm.

That night, when the meditation stopped and I sat inside my room dressed in my meditation whites, amid the fire-flies and the geckos and above the Chiang Mai city lights below, I began to think about how I hadn't realised all these angry thoughts were so pervasive. Many of them, I concluded, were petty; others did not examine the entire context of the event in question; almost all lacked perspective and empathy. None of them examined the morality of my own behavior. More than that, I realised that so many of the things I was angry about were actually in my own imagination—a kind of paranoia, or low-level psychosis was giving me an unnecessarily grim and bitter view of the world.

Mindfulness in this way, done properly, divorced from corporate goals and corporate mumbo-jumbo, can tear open your skull, and when it does you might find something that resembles a chaotic TV screen—constantly changing channels featuring random memories, future projections, fuzz, hatred, and resentment. Crystal meth didn't stop the flow—its creation of a movie-like vortex only fostered the delusion that the mind was coherent and wondrous. It is quieting the mind, not speeding it up where, perhaps, ultimate fulfillment can be found.

More meditation the next day, and while my concentration levels and impulse control made it extremely difficult for me to meditate, I noticed nonetheless a feeling of calm that, over the next few days, increased. The angry thoughts eventually just faded away. Once they started to fade away, I felt extremely clear, and I began to wonder why I had spent so long dwelling on people's bad sides—many of which were in my own imagination—that I failed to see the good in people. So after meditation, I started thinking about all the good things people had done for me, especially my parents, and I realised these far, far outweighed the bad. And when I thought of the bad things, I put them in context, and tried to think about why the people comcerned had done them, and that, like me, they had this dreadful thing called the mind which was often petty, incoherent, vain, and deeply flawed.

And I wondered, *How can I have expectations for others, when our minds are just so inherently problematic?*

I eventually chose a little temple just outside the main building and sat cross-legged in front of a 12-foot white Buddha—his body floating amid the vines and the flowers, and an elaborate crumbling cemetery behind him.

The austerity, abstinence, and ritual made my mind float, too. And the rhythm—the rhythm of the chants, rhythm of the breath, the rhythm of life and death. We are all impermanent; desire is the cause of all suffering; phenomena is unstable, transient, disenchanting.

I took a walk back to my villa, and pulled out the book I'd been reading: *Wisdom of the Buddha.*

'The body is wasted, full of sickness, and frail: this heap of corruption breaks into pieces, life indeed ends in death'.

Yes, reading was against the rules, and actually I didn't even last the full week because I was so damn hungry. But what I can tell you is that on the way out, I stared up at a pagoda as its spire pierced the sky, and I watched as the clouds floated past; I might have been a no-hoper, a fuckwit, and a cliché, I might have just been lost in delusion and lost in the self, desperate for answers after the inevitable failure of my 'chemical philosophy'—but what I felt then was a sense of the sublime.

When I returned to Chiang Mai city, in the three days after the camp, I felt so very calm and grateful, and dare I say it—*happy*. Happy as Larry, happy as a pig in shit, and I sent a few people close to me some heartfelt messages about how happy I was and how glad I was that they were in my life. Possibly they thought I had re-discovered MDMA. My mum in particular was delighted to hear from me, and I told her all about my trip, and amid the cheery small talk, I felt a sense of acceptance. *We are both deeply flawed*, I thought. The fight earlier in the year became fluid, unfrozen, it became water under the bridge—a strong bridge which had ultimately not faltered under even more trying arguments. She had, after all, put up with an awful lot from me. She was always there to help when she could.

And I needed help. The body is wasted and full of sickness. I had been using the same anti-depressants for four years by the time I got to Chiang Mai, and shortly after I left the mindfulness camp, I discovered that those anti-depressants were extremely hard to find in Thailand's northern city. After about three days without taking them—tablets designed to reduce anxiety, depression, and back pain—I felt uneasy, and had a flurry of thoughts about how unfair people had been to me. I felt my career had been a disaster, I felt panic, then despair. On one level, I knew that I was feeling this way because I had stopped taking the tablets, but my thoughts and feelings seemed so sincere. I tried mindfulness meditation, and it gave me only temporary relief. I began to wonder what value spirituality, when it seemed my 'self' was little more than a chemical reaction. I began sending out pitches to editors so full of typos and mixed up sentences that I never got a reply. The drafts of the final chapters to this book were sent back from Scribe with the message: 'I have never seen anything like this in all my years of editing.' When I looked back over them, I had long, nonsensical sentences with no punctuation that didn't mean anything. In less than a week without tablets, I faded into a dread-ridden, dreadful ghost—and in that week, other people reacted to me strangely and even street dogs, for the first time, began getting aggressive as I walked past. This was again a loss of agency, an apparent limit of freedom, and again I was dependent on my mother.

Mum ending up sending me through $500 to buy anti-depressants. Not only did I not have any money for anti-depressants, but in the ten days in total I was off them, I had screwed up nearly every professional relationship I had—at least in the short-term—and she sent me another $500 a week later, with the message 'I love you'.

There was no escaping the fact that, for better or worse, I had been taking those tablets so long they were like food or water, and without them, not even the more austere, dedicated life would make any difference.

Once that was settled, once that little piece of humility was learnt, I could concentrate on higher-order things, and the more my days wore on in Chiang Mai, the more inescapable the conclusion that 'the less I have the better I am'—self-evidently the opposite of the drug addiction ætiology of 'there is never enough'. Tablets might rescue me from despair; once that was established, there was still the pressing question of meaning, and indeed, freedom to deal with. I was finally aware what a wonderful luxury it is in life to not be bogged down by pain, misery, or poverty, and to be in a position to ask myself life's complicated spiritual questions.

I felt that the clues had been laid out for me during the mindfulness camp; mindfulness was about the joy and fulfillment of *subduing* one's mind, rather than accelerating it. It was slowing down and letting go, rather than clinging to things. I wondered about the links between a drug binge and a spiritual journey; I wondered if instead of a weekend of over-indulgence to de-clutter and start again, perhaps what I needed to do was start having weekends of austerity. Generosity is a near constant theme in Buddhism, along with morality, patience, enthusiasm, concentration, and wisdom. I already knew was it wasn't possible to experience the other or the other's need when I was on the drug. There was, I began to think, an alternative to this cycle. Trips into the netherworld of our minds could be achieved through weekends of austerity and meditation, and not through drug binges.

I was living in a cheap hotel in Chiang Mai with a TV and a bathroom. But I decided to take my austerity to another level. I went to Kathmandu, Nepal, and moved into a small room in a hostel: no TV, no Wi-Fi, no computer, no phone, and a shared bathroom (but with multiple packs of my anti-depressants).

Kathmandu is a dusty, cluttered city in a valley—it was almost purely an agricultural district a hundred years ago. It is full of Buddha and Hindu statues, and yes, suffering: poverty, stray dogs, and street people—including children who live on the sidewalk.

The suffering was difficult to digest at times; it also seemed outside of my control, and unlike the social and political problems in Australia, which obviously paled in comparison, I did not feel the same sense of being able to place cultural explanations for my own present problems. Whenever I saw the cruelty often inflicted on stray dogs and street people, I did my best to stop it. Otherwise, the problems faced by them seemed totally insurmountable, which, in the end, confirmed my ideas that empathy and compassion are lofty ideals and higher-order human and social functions.

I have to admit I liked Kathmandu because it was cheap and weird; it didn't matter how you dressed or what you looked like, and it was full of strange bookshops. I found a book called *Transcending Madness* by a Tibetan Buddhist called Chögyam Trungpa, in which he writes:

> Ego is that which is constant, it is always involved in some kind of paranoia, some kind of panic, always some kind of hope and fear. Sanity is therefore experiencing things as they are.

Trungpa draws on the Buddhist idea of the six 'Bardos' — the six realms of human existence we are continually cycling in and out of. One of the realms is the 'Hungry Ghost' realm — a source of anger, greed, ignorance, lust, envy, and pride. The Hungry Ghost means you don't want to give anything; you just take. The more you get, the more you want to receive. Ultimately, this leads to aggression, Trungpa writes, because you want to destroy anything that reminds you of giving.

However, our 'Hungry Ghost' is also useful: we should not seek to exorcise it, instead, he says we should recognise how it operates and know when we are in its realm. The Hungry Ghost can lead to two types of pain: the first is not being to achieve what you want to achieve; the second occurs once you already have your desires filled, but you have a kind of nostalgia for desire. So this second pain occurs when you are already full, but you miss being hungry — it is at that point, perhaps, you should seek to enter the world of nothingness.

Not being dominated by sour thoughts all the time gave me an increased appetite for life, and I found myself bouncing around the streets of Kathmandu in happiness most days — I had no desire to escape from my responsibility to interpet reality.

Of course, a dose of healthy cynicism dictates that my sense of liberation and happiness may merely have been the result of enjoying travel, and that these 'epiphanies' would turn to dust once I returned to my regular life in Australia, among old temptations and old friends.

I considered this, too, but it also occurred to me that I had come to pretty much what I wanted to in life. I could work full time on writing. There had been some very real economic impediments to my freedom in Australia—my career had, at the very least, stalled after having the Great Breakdown of 2008. Then I ran into conflict with my managers because of the lack of opportunity, and then I had back and neck problems that kept me out of the workforce for a long time. Combined with my reputation for being mentally unstable, the legal actions against the ABC only served to further tarnish my employment prospects, and even former peers who'd backed me stepped away. In 2009 and 2010, I had spent nearly eighteen months on unemployment benefits; I applied for jobs at a nursery and DVD store because I couldn't get a job, and even then I didn't get shortlisted. While most of my legal actions were eventually successful (I was homeless, in pain, and living on the dole in between them) I found it nearly impossible to get another job—in fact, most people at the ABC thought I was a 'disgruntled former employee' and many others believed I had been sacked. My main skill-set was in radio, and I was left high and dry and living on rice and sweet potatoes for a long time. Then my new career in law didn't turn out quite as I'd expected: first, I got low marks, which limited my career opportunities; besides which, I didn't have the temperament to be involved in litigation without a constant feeling of wanting to kill the most annoying person from the other party (or sometimes myself), and I just couldn't get excited at the prospect of a career working twelve hours a day in an oppressive office environment to have about half of my pay each week go on rent.

By 2015, though, I was writing full time and I loved it—it meant I could keep travelling around in a semi-nomadic manner, learning new things and meeting new people. And I thought, *What a wonderful thing life is!* I could choose which projects I wanted to work on, I didn't have to get up to an alarm, I didn't have annoying work colleagues I had to put up with year after year, and I had found a new direction, which, I realised, I hadn't really done since my radio career ended. I was doing what I loved every day in beautiful surrounds—it would take a hard-hearted person not to be happy.

I wondered if the great feeling I'd had when I'd left Bundaberg, about the promise of my new life emerging, hadn't been hope but intuition. In Buddhism, being paid to write, even writing itself is, I guess, what you might call an 'optimal Bardo experience'—a great experience of life, but still on a more superficial level than spirituality. The more I paid attention to my dreams, the more I noticed that, in them, I was searching for areas of missing bush land, wondering where the bush had gone, wondering what it might mean for the wildlife—and I decided to take these dreams literally, and organised with *The Good Weekend* to travel to Sumatra to spend some months writing and researching a piece on palm oil, forest fires, and deforestation.

Amid all this—and I was conscious that I'd had many 'big ideas' when I left rehab in 2008—I had lived through my longest period of not having any amphetamines since my drug-free spell from 2002 to 2006. Never smoking pot again would be my next goal.

I met several inspiring young Australian men, all in their early twenties, who were in Nepal to volunteer: young men who seemed to know already what it had taken me thirty-five years to learn—the value of selflessness. They knew I was gay, and they didn't treat me in any way differently in the slightest. It was about then that I decided that Buddhism had helped me a lot, but to call myself a Buddhist and fully adopt a Buddhist way of life was not quite for me—many cultural Buddhists meditate from a very young age, and I concluded that we can learn from Buddhism, but ultimately, unless you become a monk, it is designed for eastern cultures and people who have developed a unique space in their mind to experience its teachings.

As the year wore on, research into use and abuse of crystal meth in the community would foster a mixed message. A National Drug and Alcohol Research Centre drug survey about crystal-meth use released in October 2015 would reveal that the drug had more or less stabilised in use among most drug populations, except for intravenous drug users, who had increased their crystal-meth use by six per cent between 2014 and 2015. The survey also showed that among people who used traditional 'party drugs' like MDMA as well as crystal meth were also cutting down, albeit slightly, on their crystal meth use. NDARC researchers concluded that users who are younger, university educated, and unlikely to have a prison history were the ones cutting down; for the most serious drug users, though, use was going up.

There were also some trials in Australia by the end of 2015 into the use of two drugs—naltrexone and N-acetylcysteine—to help people wean off crystal meth.

And then, in December 2015, the Turnbull government announced a $300 million plan to combat crystal meth. The vast bulk of the money—$241 million—was dedicated to treatment, and would be administered through Australia's newly created 31 Primary Health Networks (bureaucratically organised areas of primary health care around Australia). These primary health networks would be given discretion about how they spend this money. Additionally, new money was given to doctors, and specialists would also be paid $13 million to treat ice users with a new Medicare payment to increase the availability of treatment.

$24 million was dedicated to 'help families and communities by providing the resources, information and support they need to respond to ice', and $18.8 million was allocated to setting up a new Centre for Clinical Excellence for Emerging Drugs of Concern.

Just $16 million of the $300 million package was dedicated to law enforcement, including $5 million for the Australian Crime Commission to deploy officers internationally, and $10 million, taken from the proceeds-of-crime fund, to 'inform the design and development of a National Criminal Intelligence System and enhance our ability to share intelligence with state and territory partners'.

In the week following the announcement, the government almost universally approved the ice plan: St Vincent's Health Australia CEO, Toby Hall told *The Guardian* Australia: 'The government has clearly listened to the taskforce and those working on the front line of the problem.' The same article quoted the head of the Public Health Association of Australia, Michael Moore: 'This announcement marks the first steps in a sensible return to realign funding, focus and efforts into moving away from a largely prohibitionist approach to the much more effective approach of harm minimisation.' Matt Noffs, chief executive of the Noffs Foundation and part of the ice taskforce consultations, told Fairfax Media it was Ken Lay who supplied the 'oxygen' that Malcolm Turnbull needed to take a 'giant step forward'.

Noffs would later tell Fairfax Media he didn't think $250 million was enough, and it could potentially mean that less than a quarter of the staff members required would be funded. Other concerns expressed by groups such as the Australian Medical Association and providers of alcohol and drug treatment included whether or not the primary health networks would spend the money appropriately, and whether or not they have should have been given the money to begin with.

When the Liberal National Party Abbott government was elected in 2013, one of the first things it did was defund the Australian Drug and Alcohol Commission Alcohol and Other Drugs Council of Australia (ADCA) — so the body no longer exists. The council was Australia's peak body for organisations working to minimise the harm caused by drugs and alcohol, and had an annual budget of $1.6 million from the federal health department. The council ran the public awareness 'Drug week' campaign, which also no longer exists. From 2002 to 2005, Australia also had a National School Drug Education Program, but it was dismantled in 2007. In her 20-year timeline of Australian drug policy, Dr Caitlin Hughes pointed out that drug-crime related asset seizures are put into general revenue rather than put back into spend for tackling the drug problem:

> The Federal Government announced that from 1 July 2012 it would return all money from its Confiscated Assets Account (an estimated $58.3 million over four years) to consolidated revenue. Since 2002 proceeds of crime has been a key source of funding crime prevention initiatives, drug treatment provision, illicit drug diversion programs and law enforcement projects such as DUMA & the development of an Enhanced National Intelligence Picture on Illicit Drugs.

This move already puts Australia at odds with the New Zealand approach, which uses forfeited funds to help problematic drug users.

Despite these criticisms, there is no doubt the federal government's plan — which is the result of appointing Ken Lay as taskforce chief under the Abbott government — is a surprisingly progressive one. It should also be remembered that Ritter's 2011 study showed the total state and federal government funding for drug treatment was just $361 million—an additional $250 million to provide treatment for one drug is nothing to be sneezed at. Given the status quo and the weight of public opinion, it was not without risk for the federal government to follow expert advice on creating a new crystal-meth policy. At the same time, it is consistent with a nation that has been flexible, relatively sensible (often despite the rhetoric), and effective with drug policy at a federal level. It remains an ongoing issue, however, that our state and territory governments continue to run with populist law-and-order lines rather than evidence-based policy in dealing with a range of social problems—including illicit drug use.

Tellingly, the federal government's emphasis on treatment was received reasonably well by Australia's right-wing tabloids. The *Herald Sun* even published an opinion piece by Alan Tudge, assistant minister to the prime minister:

> The executive director of the United Nations Office on Drugs and Crime stated in 2007 that societies have the drug problem that they deserve … Australia deserves better than being seen as the biggest ice users. Our ice plan will hopefully be the start of that change.

It is, of course, perfectly possible that crystal meth will come and go; emerge, linger, disappear, and then come again. Although, its lesson is surely that the next heavy drug to come along will almost certainly be wholly synthetic—perhaps even another variation on the methamphetamine formula.

And Australia's crystal-meth problem has, if nothing else, shown the gaps in the dominant-to-date policy approach. It has also provided new challenges to both treatment providers, and users and abusers of party drugs. It seems, for the most part, that drug policy in Australia is turning in the direction that drug policy experts say it should be going. While rehabs and drug counselling centres are still citing long waiting lists, there is hope that with the federal government emphasis on treatment, more of the people who are struggling with crystal meth will find the resources they need.

Life can be mundane once you stop dreaming; many recovering crystal-meth addicts may find that waking life calls them to examine themselves in challenging and exciting ways that they have never imagined before.

For me, crystal meth set into place thinking patterns that were often exaggerations of myself, and our culture, at its worst, and what is particularly hard to recognise is the way in which these linger afterwards. For many months after, even long after the cravings have passed, the ways of seeing I developed on crystal meth continued, and continued in a way that was not only hard for me to notice—because I was in the midst of them—but also because they were magnifications of things already in my personality. This made it extremely difficult for others around me to notice as well. I can be self-absorbed, self-victimising, nasty, suspicious, grandiose, owned by ambition, manipulative, reckless, and extremely judgemental of others. Ice made this worse, but it was already within me.

It also became obvious to me after seven months after I stopped using how little shame I had for my own transgressions—I had, in a sense, been walking around naked during and after the addiction—and unabashedly so. But I also can't help but wonder whether I needed to tear off my old clothes, and go into the depths of madness to see where my life and self were lacking. It was only through this process, and then through coming to a resolution about how to be completely abstinent, that the lack of meaning in my life and my deepest callings became clear.

Drug-treatment programs are there to show you how you can stop using drugs and find other ways to enjoy life—however, I think many of us in recovery need to realise that there is more to life than mere pleasure.

Carl Jung published 40 books on psychoanalysis before he died in 1961. *The Red Book*, a notebook of Jung's inner experiences, was not released to the public until 2009. These notebooks were written over a period of roughly sixteen years, starting in his late thirties just before the Second World War. After his death, the family refused to allow these notebooks to be published—Jung had never wanted the books published during his lifetime, and there are some perfectly legitimate reasons for that. Jung was worried his notebooks would destroy his credibility; in his own words, he wondered if he was 'menaced by a psychosis' or 'doing schizophrenia'. The select few people who saw his notebooks, stored in a vault in Switzerland after his death, often regarded them as the work of a psychotic.

The notebook that would become *The Red Book* first began when Jung began to face a kind of inexplicable lack in his experience of life. He had started to feel that his life was in some kind of spiritual crisis—that he had lost his soul.

Jung, a prolific daydreamer, began fantasising about digging a hole in the ground. As he kept imagining, he found that these fantasies took on a life of their own; as he dug deeper and deeper into this imaginary hole in the ground, he eventually reached a strange, self-perpetuating symbolic land.

Intrigued by what he found, he began practising this descent into the imaginary underworld each night. Soon after, he began recording what this world presented, and when his journal was finally taken out of a Swiss vault at the turn of the new millennium, it would be filled with intricate drawings of strange serpentine beasts with dozens of legs, encounters with old mystics in castles, winged humans, mandalas, and sea monsters. He writes that he travelled to the 'Land of the Dead', where magnanimous plots developed. He described his visions as coming in an 'incessant stream' as a result of deliberately switching off his unconscious.

Jung later wrote that he felt he had travelled the same borderlands as both great artists and lunatics; he knew that he had to let himself 'plummet down into them'. Throughout these experiences, a female figure resurfaces—she tells him not to fear madness but to accept it, even to tap into it as a source of creativity. 'If you want to find paths, you should also not spurn madness, since it makes up such a great part of your nature.'

Just prior to sinking into these depths, Jung felt that he had accomplished everything he had ever set out to do in the world: professional success, fame, marriage, children, wealth, prestige, etc. He felt that what he was doing in these imaginary experiences was going deep into the underground of his unconscious, and it was here that he rediscovered meaning in his life, and a kind of collective meaning in all human life. He felt that going into the dark allowed him to find the things that were missing from his consciousness, and he was able to integrate them; by doing so, he restored meaning to his life.

The most recent photo I saw of Smithy was a picture of him with his new, young girlfriend who lay, smirking, sticking up her middle finger as Smithy slept like a dead man, with his sickly, grey skin and marks on his face. By some reports, he was now easing off the meth and taking GHB—a cheaper, less exhausting drug—regularly instead. He was moved on by the landlord from his place in Pakenham—that house in the Toomuc Valley—and eventually he lost contact with everybody who knew him. I don't know where he ended up or what became of him.

Twelve months after the order giving custody of the twins to Smithy's father and stepmother, the Children's Court would make an order for the boys to stay with them indefinitely. It was hard not to conclude that, all things considered, it was the best choice of several bad options.

Beck has given up crystal meth, though. She's worked in some odd jobs as a waitress and a food server. She has remained living with her parents, and settled into a long-term relationship with a mechanic who lived interstate — a man she met on a dating app.

Other than that, I don't know the details of how she lives her life. By calling the Child Protection Unit, I knew that was the end of the friendship. Eighteen months after I left the house, Beck and I still haven't spoken. This, I have to admit, makes me feel incredibly relieved. I wonder how much I went back to Beck again and again out of habit, out of a drug habit, and also to make sure the kids were being looked after properly. I wonder if we actually had anything in common other than our drug use, born in that cold valley together in a state of teenage-angst isolation. I decided to cut contact with most of her family — all of them, except for Hayley.

Hayley finished Year 11; she had no specific plans about what to do. However, she told me she was determined to make something big of her life. She stayed living with a family in an area right near her high school. Two years had passed by this stage, and she still hadn't spoken a word to her mum. She still spoke with other members of the family — her aunties and Beck's parents — but she never saw them. She smoked cigarettes for a little while and then quit. She told me that she drinks only sometimes. She jogs most days, and eats a very salad-heavy diet. She takes vitamins every day. The last photo I saw of her, she was in her school uniform, flashing her teeth, holding up two fingers with a caption saying 'I love education'.

I keep waiting for the cracks to appear, but they don't. Perhaps they already did, and, as they say, that's how the light got in.

# Select bibliography

## Books

Alexander, A. and Roberts, M. *High Culture: reflections on addiction and modernity* (2003)

Allsop, S. and Lee, N. (eds) *Perspectives on amphetamine-type stimulants* (2012)

Andreasen, N. *The Creative Brain: the science of genius* (2006)

Andrews, M. *Narrative Imagination and Everyday Life* (2014)

Armstrong, K. *Buddha* (2001)

Burroughs, B. *Speed* (1970)

Burroughs, W. *Junkie* (1953)

Burroughs, W. *Naked Lunch* (1959)

Burrows, D., Flaherty, B., and MacAvoy, M. *Illicit psychostimulant use in Australia* (1993)

Csikszentmihalyi, M. *Flow: the psychology of optimal experience* (1990)

Dick, P. *A Scanner Darkly* (1997)

Eigen, M. *The Psychotic Core* (1986)

Fletcher, A. *Inside Rehab: the surprising truth about addiction treatment — and how to get help that works* (2013)

Fraser, S. and Moore, D. (eds) *The Drug Effect: health, crime and society* (2013)

Hart, C. *High Price: a neuroscientist's journey of self-discovery that challenges everything you know about drugs and society* (2013)

Jung, C. *Man and His Symbols* (1964)

Jung, C. *The Red Book* (2009)

Kaufman, W. *Existentialism from Dostoevsky to Sartre* (1956)

Khantzian, E. *Treating Addiction as Human Process* (2007)

Klee, H. *Amphetamine Misuse: international perspectives on current trends* (1996)

Kleinman, M., Caulkins, J., and Hawken, A. *Drugs and Drug Policy: what everyone needs to know* (2011)

Knox, M. *Scattered: the inside story of ice in Australia* (2008)

Lewis, M. *Memoirs of an Addicted Brain: a neuroscientist examines his former life on drugs* (2011)

Lewis, M. *The Biology of Desire: why addiction is not a disease* (2015)

Moore, D. and Dietze, P. (eds) *Drugs and Public Health: Australian perspectives on policy and practice* (2013)

Muller, M. *Wisdom of the Buddha: the unabridged Dhammapada* (2000)

Owen, F. *No Speed Limit: the highs and lows of meth* (2008)

Rasmussen, N. *On Speed: the many lives of amphetamine* (2008)

Reding, N. *Methland: the death and life of an American small town* (2009)

Ritter A., King T., and Hamilton, M. (ed.) *Drug Use in Australian Society* (2013)

Sartre, J. *Age of Reason: a novel* (1945)

Sharp, J. *Quitting Crystal Meth: What to Expect & What to Do: a handbook for the first year of recovery from crystal methamphetamine* (2013)

Trungpa, C. *Transcending Madness: the experience of the six Bardos* (1992)

Weisheit, R. and White, W. *Methamphetamine: its history, pharmacology, and treatment* (2009)

# Journal Articles

Bousman, C., McKetin, R., and Burns, R. 'Typologies of positive psychotic symptoms in methamphetamine dependence', *The American Journal on Addictions*, Online Early Version, pp. 1–4 (2014)

Green, R. and Moore, D. '"Meth circles" and "pipe pirates": crystal methamphetamine smoking and identity management among a social network of young adults', *Substance Use and Misuse*, 48, (2013)

Hall, W. and Hando, J. 'Route of administration and adverse effects of amphetamine use among young adults in Sydney, Australia', *Drug and Alcohol Review*, vol. 13, no. 3, pp. 277–284 (1994)

Hides, L., Dawe, S., and McKetin, R. 'Primary and substance-induced psychotic disorders in methamphetamine users', *Psychiatry Research*, vol. 226, pp. 91–96 (2014)

Lee, N., Harney, A., and Pennay, A. 'Examining the temporal relationship between methamphetamine use and mental health comorbidity', *Advances in Dual Diagnosis*, vol. 5, no. 1, pp. 23–31 (2012)

McKetin, R., Lubman, D., and Najman, J. 'Does methamphetamine use increase violent behaviour? Evidence from a prospective longitudinal study', *Addiction*, vol. 109, no. 5 (2014)

McKetin, R., Lubman, D., and Baker, A. 'Dose-related psychotic symptoms in chronic methamphetamine users: evidence from a prospective longitudinal study', *JAMA Psychiatry*, vol. 70, no. 3, pp. 319–324 (2013)

Thomson, N. and Moore, D. 'Methamphetamine "facts": the production of a "destructive" drug in Australian scientific texts. *Addiction Research & Theory*, vol. 22, no. 6, pp. 451–462 (2014)

Weatherburn, D., Jones, C., Snowball, L., and Hua 'The NSW Drug Court: a re-evaluation of its effectiveness', *Crime and Justice Bulletin*, no. 121, Bureau of Crime Statistics and Research (2008)

## Reports and Government Publications

Australian Crime Commission, Australian Illicit Drug Data Report(s) 2002–03 to 2013–14, inclusive

Australian Crime Commission, *Organised Crime in Australia* (2013)

Australian Crime Commission 'Clandestine laboratories and precursors', *Crime Profile Series* (2013)

Australian Crime Commission 'Amphetamine-type stimulants', *Crime Profile Series* (2013)

Australian Crime Commission, *Outlaw Motorcycle Gangs Fact Sheet* (2013)

Coyne, J., White, V., and Alvarez, C. *Methamphetamine: Focusing Australia's National Ice Strategy on the problem, not the symptoms* (2015)

Department of the Prime Minister and Cabinet, *Final Report of the National Ice Taskforce* (2015)

Global Commission on Drug Policy, *War on Drugs: Report of the Global Commission on Drug Policy* (2011)

Law Reform, Drugs and Crime Prevention, *Parliament of Victoria Committee Inquiry into the Supply and Use of Methamphetamines, Particularly Ice in Victoria, Parts 1 and 2* (2014)

Ministerial Council on Drug Strategy National Drug Strategy 2010–15. *A framework for action on alcohol, tobacco and other drugs* (2011)

Ritter, A., Lancaster, K., Grech, K., and Reuter, P. *An assessment of illicit drug policy in Australia (1985 to 2010): themes and trends*, National Drug and Alcohol Research Centre, University of New South Wales, Sydney, Australia (2011)

Roxburgh, A.D., Ritter, A., Slade, T., and Burns, L. *Trends in Drug Use and Related Harms in Australia, 2001 to 2013*, National Drug and Alcohol Research Centre, University of New South Wales, Sydney (2014)

Roxburgh, A.D., Ritter, A., Grech, K., Slade, T., and Burns, L. *Trends in Drug Use and Related Harms in Australia, 2001 to 2011*, Drug

Policy Modelling Program, National Drug and Alcohol Research
Centre, University of New South Wales (2011)
United Nations Office on Drugs and Crime (UNODC) 2013b,
*Transnational Organised Crime in East Asia and the Pacific*
United Nations Office on Drugs and Crime (UNODC) World Drug
Report(s) 1999–2015 inclusive

# Acknowledgements

It's difficult to know where to start, quite frankly. Thanks to Erik Jensen for taking a risk by publishing the article detailing my crystal-meth addiction in *The Saturday Paper*, and huge thanks to Scribe for taking an even bigger risk by agreeing to publish this book. The editors at Scribe have been patient, flexible, open-minded, and very kind from the very start. Thank you. And thanks to my agent, Shelia Drummond, for making this all happen for me.

There are some others I would like to single out who have been particularly helpful to my media career in a variety of ways: Steve Cannane, Rosie Beaton, Kyla Slaven, Ben Naparstek, Justine Kelly, Vicki Kerrigan, Serpil Senelmis, John Safran, Lauren Martin, Jo Curtin, and Jennifer Hopper.

Thanks to Mrs Haywood, my Year 11 literature teacher, who introduced me to T.S. Eliot, and to Philipa Rothfield at La Trobe University for introducing me to Georges Bataille and Julia Kristeva. Thanks to Vicky G. for introducing me to William Burroughs when I was a 19-year-old meth junkie and philosophy student.

Thanks to my parents, and my life-long friends Bree, Erika, and John. Thanks, in general, to everyone for putting up with me.